—THE—
FOREVER
FAT BURNER

THE SECRET TO OPTIMIZING YOUR HEALTH, LONGEVITY, AND BODY COMPOSITION

Linné Linder, N.D.

1st Edition

Disclaimer: It is possible that for some of you reading this, medically-assisted weight loss may be an important avenue for you. If so, it would be wise to talk to a practitioner who specializes in weight loss with a well-rounded, safe, and holistic approach. Look for a licensed practitioner that will review of your hormones, blood chemistry, stress levels, sleep habits, potential sensitivities/allergies to foods, liver detoxification pathways, etc. In fact, it is wise, when deciding to lose weight that you have these areas assessed to rule out any metabolic dysfunction or road blocks that may be preventing your weight from shifting. It is fairly common for some individuals who eat healthily and exercise to get stuck at an overweight or obese set point because of metabolic and hormone imbalance. Usually, when this is the case, *no* diet or exercise tips or tricks will facilitate improvement, unless one addresses the underlying issues. The program that I have outlined in this book is intended to assist those who are metabolically sound; do not require significant detoxification assistance; understand their food sensitivities or have been tested for them and have hormone levels and adrenal functioning, all within *reasonable* limits.

This book is not meant to diagnose or treat any health condition and is information-based only. The author is not rendering medical advice, nor is the book intended to diagnose, prescribe or treat any disease, condition or illness. You should seek medical clearance from a licensed physician before starting this or any nutrition and exercise program. The author and publisher claim no responsibility to any person or entity for any liability, loss or damage caused (directly or indirectly) as a result of the application of concepts in this book.

Now that the necessary legal speak is out of the way, I highly advise that you see a holistic practitioner who can assist you in assessing these areas before embarking on any new dietary program (especially if you have had frustrating plateaus or stubborn weight gain, despite your efforts). With the combination of the necessary screening tests, nutraceutical supplementation, and hormone assistance, I have seen remarkable changes in the health and lives of many people. It would be an honor and a privilege to assist you.

Also, it is important to note, that while my background is in science, this book is not meant to be a discussion on research or the science behind my findings or the conclusions of others. Rather, it is intended to be a quick, concise guide to helping you find your rhythm and your ideal healthful body. Likewise, my goal is to assist you to make wise choices when it comes to food, self-talk, and exercise. Where applicable, please research topics you are interested in, on your own, and make appropriate determinations based on the scientific studies you find. I would advise you to steer clear of opinions and fads and take a look at clinical, non-biased, double-blind, peer-reviewed studies. I am *not* asking you to take my word for it. However, I have done a lot of research for myself over the years and thus, have created a condensed version of my findings for you to use as a starting point in your lifestyle journey. Where it is deemed appropriate, I have referenced these influences and resources. It is equally important to note that my findings are a result of the knowledge and wisdom from many experts, many authors, many scientists, many bloggers, many mentors and many of my successes and failures. Without these influences, this book would never have been possible.

I dedicate this book to all those

who inspired its creation:

To my parents, Ron and Lyn, who have always supported my desire to achieve more, to be more and to dream more. Thank you for always believing in me.

To my in-laws, Marty and Sue, who have been an anchor of wisdom, encouragement, and support through life's trials and tribulations.

To my sister, Kari, who is a cheerleader by nature and a rather talented young woman.

To my patients who have entrusted me to join them in their health journey and who have provided the feedback and experience that inspired the pages of this book.

To my husband, John, who is my rock, the best PR Manager and my best friend who knows all of my dirty bits and loves me anyway. You are God's greatest gift.

To my friend, Bob, who believed in me when I could not see my potential and who provided the mentorship and leadership skills that helped me to bloom where planted. I treasure this mentorship, to this day. We weathered the trenches together and went through hell and made it through to tell about it. You will never know the lasting treasure of impact that you have had on my life.

To the dream that one day, preventative care and holistic medicine will, once again, become "standard." To the dream that natural medicine will be promoted by our government's healthcare system as a means of naturally deflating the cost of healthcare. To the dream that, in following these principles, the obesity rate and inflammatory disease processes that are rampant in the United States will dramatically decrease.

To the continuing hope that our society, as a whole, will jump off all dietary bandwagons and avoid all fads and work toward rediscovering how to investigate the root cause of weight gain (and reverse it). To the continuing hope that we will accomplish this by employing customized, individualized approaches, recognizing hormonal and metabolic individuality.

Table of Contents

A Note to the Reader:
Introduction to the Last Diet Book You'll Ever Own

Everyone is looking for a quick fix or a golden ticket to a healthy and fit body. However, it is the quick fixes that—while they can produce results—are not sustainable, nor enjoyable in the long run. In fact, most diets never get to the heart of why your body gains or lets go of weight. The problem is that the model of calories in and calories out; eat less food and exercise to lose weight, only works temporarily and is not sustainable long-term for most people. Besides, this model often leads to metabolic dysfunction and unfavorable set points that are often higher than when one started dieting. The reason for this is that the underlying issue of hormone regulation is what should be the focus. The food we eat, how often we eat and the exercise we engage in, all affect our body's ability to burn or to store fat. I'll dive a bit deeper into the everyday players of metabolism in a later chapter; but, for now, know that your inability to burn fat has more to do with your hormones than with how well you eat or exercise. I see this scenario in my clinical experience, often. In fact, I see it often enough that I was inspired to write this book to help the masses with what has become a dilemma for over half of our population.

The goal of this nutrition guide is to create a customizable plan — that while you are adapting to this new lifestyle (and it must be a way of life), you don't feel deprived. The trick is to enjoy the process and celebrate the successes, no matter how seemingly small or insignificant. For example, your goal may be to lose 20 pounds. And, chances are, you are going to accomplish that purpose if you follow this plan correctly; but, you will also accomplish other things that deserve just as much of your attention and just as much celebration. You may lower your blood pressure. You may lose your sugar cravings and loosen the bonds that a carbohydrate addiction has had on you. You may find it easier to climb stairs. You may increase your "good" (HDL) cholesterol. You may get sick less often, if at all. You may experience less joint pain. My point is, that should your weight loss stall temporarily (and this is natural), keep track of the health improvements and markers that may not be as apparent as a change in the scale.

So, now that we know that we can expect some great results, what does this plan entail? It is quite simple: you are going to learn how to eat whole foods, in the proper portions, the correct amount and at the appropriate intervals. That's it. We can all go home now. But seriously, it is not a complicated process. However, we have made it so with all of the confusing diets, get-thin-quick books, pills, supplements, and bombardment of advertisements for weight loss. In the next few pages, I will outline how you can see through the bull and get down to what has been a proven method for ultimate fat loss and ultimate health: *not* with dieting and over-exercising but by balancing your hormonal *response* to food and exercise.

I will help you determine how many calories you should be getting and how to adjust this number to suit your needs and your fitness level. In fact, the calorie estimate is exactly that: an estimate. Once you get a feel for what foods to eat and the serving sizes, you will *not* have to count calories. It will be as easy as checking off a box and tracking how many servings you get each day, to ensure a well-rounded nutrition profile. Surprisingly, fat loss is not always about counting calories. But more on that, later.

Also, I'll help you with your grocery shopping, meal prep and give you some simple recipes to get you started. I've even added some printable sheets for you to use if you are a visual person who needs lists to refer to (all located in one place at journeytowardjoy.com under the Resources tab). But wait! There's more! I've included Progress Tracking Sheets, Workout Sheets, Macronutrient Calculator Sheets, etc. for those who like to have these types of guides handy.

It is important to note that if you haven't done so already, please get tested for food allergies and sensitivities. Any foods that you are eating that you are sensitive to or allergic to are creating an immune response in your gut—and thus, are preventing you from decreasing inflammation, improving digestion, losing weight, regulating hormones, calming your immune system, etc. Ultimately, food allergens prevent you from obtaining optimum health. Once you discover these foods, you may choose to eliminate them from the recipes or shopping lists, in this book. Feel free to research alternative options.

This diet is a lower carbohydrate, a higher fat diet that has withstood the test of time. Our ancestors did not have access to all of the sugars, processed carbohydrates, chemicals, hormones and toxins that are abundant in our food, today. The health benefits of eating quality fats, meats, fish, poultry, vegetables, nuts, seeds and some fruits have been proven to assist the body in optimizing overall health. In fact eating in this manner—while counter intuitive, given our current food pyramid, FDA requirements, American Heart Association and American Diabetes Association recommendations, a higher fat and lower carbohydrate diet continues to blow these suggested dietary guidelines out of the water. People who adopt a whole foods-centered, high fat and lower carb lifestyle can expect to experience incredible health benefits over time. But, you don't have to take my word for it.

Why is this the case? Why does a grain-free diet, low in carbohydrates and high in fat produce incredible health benefits? You see, sugar creates a lot of metabolic waste and free radicals when it is being broken down and utilized by our cells mitochondria (the power house of our cells). Conversely, fat produces an efficient and clean source of energy in your body (think diesel truck vs. an electric car). By eating higher fat and keeping your carbohydrates low, the body undergoes what we call mitochondrial biogenesis, meaning that our cells produce more mitochondria when in a state of ketosis (using the metabolic breakdown of fat for fuel). Fat creates not only cleaner fuel but produces more energy with less waste. Your body becomes the Tesla amongst a sea of Ford trucks. I do not intend to offend my Ford-truck-driving friends. I'm just trying to help you understand the potential that your physiology is capable of with this transition.

What is the result of this mitochondrial miracle occurring in your cells? Your cells age more slowly and experience an enhanced quality of life. What?!? Yes, you read correctly. By avoiding sugar and certain carbohydrates, you prevent glycation; sugar attaching to proteins in the body. This process is called AGES or advanced glycation end products. However, there is little glycation in a lower-carb, higher-fat diet. For example, age spots on the skin are a reflection of oxidization and inflammation of skin cells. When there is less glycation, good things can get in the cell, and bad things can get out, rather easily. If the cell is unhealthy, cell death (or apoptosis) happens quicker with less glycation. Who doesn't want to age slower?

Moreover, fat is insulin neutral. It will not cause any increase in blood sugar — and thus, will not cause the pancreas to secrete insulin. It is important to note that in the presence of insulin, even a little, the body will not burn fat. However, if we can provide the body with enough dense nutrition that is insulin neutral, and in the proper amounts, the body will turn toward burning fat as its primary fuel source —either the food we take in or our body's fat stores! How exciting is that! In essence, you become a fat burning machine.

Also, this type of eating will naturally help to alleviate autoimmune conditions, down-regulate inflammation, reduce pain and significantly reduce symptoms seen in chronic diseases. You may build more lean body tissue, burn more fat and reduce cravings. You may also experience improved mental alertness and clarity, as well as mood stabilization and increased energy. As a bonus side effect, you may notice improved skin tone and color, more soft skin, less saggy skin...and the list of benefits continues. Now, do you understand why I am so excited to have implemented this way of eating into my own life? This diet will not only preserve lean muscle tissue but help you to become a lean, mean, fat burning machine.

Now, before we dive into the details of the program, you should know that there are variations to fit every body type. You see, not everyone will thrive on the same amount of fruit servings or complex carbohydrate servings per day. Some people will feel incredible and see amazing results from cutting out fruit and complex carbohydrates, altogether. Others may benefit from a little fruit while some folks may take advantage of a couple of servings of fruit and a couple of servings of complex carbohydrates per day. In this book, I provide the parameters for you and teach you how to gauge *your* body's response to food and how to adjust the servings according to where *you* are at in the process and how *you* feel.

You probably have a lot of questions and are wondering how on earth to get started. Never fear, I will guide you. However, before you embark on the best healthful habits of your life, we are going to need to get some *esse*ntial foundation laid. You can't drive an unbuilt Tesla. First, we are going to have to put all the necessary parts together to ensure that you will enjoy driving your car for the rest of your life and be successful doing so.

How to Read This Book: I want you to think of this book more as a resource guide, than as something you need to read cover to cover. You will find several chapters that you refer to more often than others. Definitely start with **Section I** before you read **Section II**. These two sections will be the most important parts for you to navigate through.

Section I of this book is an introduction to the diet and exercise plan that I have created for you. In these chapters, you will build the appropriate foundation for success for this program (or any program for that matter). Make sure you determine if you are a "high carb" or a "low carb" person and walk through the guidelines provided to prepare you for **The Plan** in **Section II**.

Section II is really the core of your new program. You will refer to these chapters often. Chapter 8 outlines your new food list and how to choose the best options. Chapter 9 helps you calculate your caloric needs and serving requirements. This chapter also provides all of the fine-tuning you will need to customize your diet based upon hormonal responses to food, eating habits and exercise.

Chapter 10 outlines the basics of your workout program and how to simplify what you may be currently doing. You can further customize your exercise routine to fit your needs and to address your goals.

Section III is your guide to further customize your program. This part of the book should not be read first and should only be a reference tool, if you have tried The Plan as outlined for a minimum of two months. However, you can refer to the Daily Detoxification and Breaking the Plateau chapters at any time you deem necessary. These two chapters are brimming with helpful information.

Section IV is your resource guide. This includes all of my own recipes that I use on a regular basis. I've added a **Resources** section that lists all the DVDs, online workouts, books, apps, etc. that have helped shape my current regimen or that I find useful.

Throughout the pages of this book I have peppered in "TIPS" that provide fun information that I have curated for you.

Well, that about sums it up! Are you ready? Good. If you are willing to commit to the process, then I am excited to commit to assisting you every step of the way.

Now, before we get started, I think you should know that you are not alone in your struggles. In the following pages, I want to share my journey and why I am so passionate about helping you with yours.

Let's get started!

PART 1
LAYING THE GROUNDWORK

Chapter 1

My Weight Loss Journey
(Why I Wrote This Book for You)

The Beginning of My Journey

As a child, I was a relatively active and fit. I played outside at every opportunity I could find. I remember weighing in at 96 pounds in the 6th grade. I ate whatever I wanted including lots of white bread with peanut butter and jelly. My favorite meals were school lunches (remember the hot dogs wrapped in bread?) with chocolate milk. My parents weren't big fans of cooking back then. Both of my parents worked hard, and my mom was going to night school for her MBA so, as a result, we often ate out at fast food restaurant chains. Now don't get me wrong. My parents cooked homemade meals that were relatively "healthy"; but, a lot of nutrition-related knowledge has changed since I was in grade school. Back then, it was common knowledge that diet coke and fat-free cookies were "healthy." I'll save any outbursts on the dangers of these food items, for another time.

Interestingly enough, when I reached junior high, I continued to eat the same, and with the help of puberty and fun hormone bursts, I grew taller and significantly wider. I recall purchasing size 13/14 jeans back then. Junior high wasn't pleasant for me as sometimes the popular kids would make comments about my backside and how big it was. I remember being embarrassed to take my clothes off in the locker room for gym class. I maintained this weight and size through high school—and thankfully, the bullying comments ceased in the new environment. When I reached college, I made an effort to walk every day and to research every diet I could find. I tried high protein, low carbohydrate. I tried high carbohydrate, low protein. I tried vegan. I tried vegetarian. I tried Atkins. I tried The Zone. I tried EVERYTHING! And yes, I did lose some weight and got down to 137 pounds with a high carbohydrate low-fat approach; but, I could not maintain my new weight because I was *always* hungry.

The Journey Continues

Then I headed off to graduate school, and despite the year-long nutrition course I took, I still did not know how to eat. I continued searching for the perfect fitness and nutrition plan. I joined a gym and worked out two hours a day, six days a week. I killed myself attempting to enlist the guidance of a trainer. I did every class the gym had to offer and lifted weights. I tried eating only whole foods. I tried eating six times a day. I exhausted every fitness program and eating plan. I even signed up for a 103-mile cycling race, to get fit. Despite all of this, I remained a tight size 12, 170 pounds and frustrated with my lack of progress.

At some point, I gave up my gym membership for financial reasons (I was a poor college student) and invested in some Pilates DVDs and followed a strict 1200 calorie diet. I went from 170 pounds to 140 pounds in a few months. I finally felt comfortable in my skin as a 5'9" tall women. And while this was a great accomplishment for me, I stayed at or around this weight (+ 5 pounds) for 11 years. After a while, I felt that I still could achieve a greater fitness level and a better body composition. It wasn't until my gut was chronically bloated from inflammation and dysbiosis (overgrowth of the wrong gut bugs) that I felt determined to search out new options.

My friend Mary (Healing Cave Lady) introduced me to the Paleo diet to get my gut healthy (for excellent recipes and a wealth of info, check out her website here). It helped a little at first; but, I didn't see results in my waistline until I started minimizing carbohydrates. Even on the Paleo diet, I found myself overeating plantains, sweet potatoes, beets, etc. in place of the grains I had given up. Once I started watching my carbohydrate intake, a shift occurred. I continued to eat whole foods and to consume lots of quality fat, proteins, and vegetables. I began to see changes with the scale and with my body. Mostly, I was following a more Primal Blueprint diet and was able to get down to 140 pounds again.

The Infamous Plateau

But shortly after my progress, the infamous "plateau" struck and struck hard. While I felt better (I stopped getting sick; my itchy skin issues went away; my abdomen was firmer and flatter, etc.), I still was in pursuit of the losing the last "vanity pounds" so to speak. I was a healthy size 6-8; but, I wanted to push my fitness boundaries. I had just turned 40 years old, and I wanted to be in the *best* shape of my life. I wanted to continue to enjoy my favorite "cheat foods" without starving. I wanted a challenging workout that didn't make me curse at my television. I wanted all of this while continuing to see progress. It sounds nearly impossible, right?

Breaking the Plateau

I did some research on portion control and found ranges that fitness experts recommend. I started tracking my caloric intake and keeping my daily range within a healthy, but effective level. I did not give up dark chocolate, red wine, and artisan cheeses. I picked an exercise program that I thought would challenge me and help me improve flexibility, strength, and endurance. I kept a tally sheet of my portions and kept my calories and carbohydrates under control. I ate more protein and more vegetables. I ate a little less fat and tracked my workouts and my progress. I chose to cook as much of my food as possible. Suddenly, my plateau was busted. My weight started dropping. And dropping. And dropping.

Overall, I have continued to see progress in my strength, muscle definition, and overall body composition. Yes, it has taken me 20 years to figure out what works for me. Yes, it has been frustrating—and at times, I have given up on my routine (more than once or twice). Regardless, my goals remain steadfast: to become the best version of myself that I can create —and in doing so, to share with you, all the tips, tricks, and recipes that I have found the most useful in my journey toward losing 45+ pounds. My goal is to assist you if weight loss and improved fitness are part of your journey, too.

Just a few months after this decision to push my fitness level, I easily dropped 15 more pounds of fat, my size two jeans were loose on me, and I became the leanest I have ever been in my life. I continue to see progress to this day. Please do not misunderstand me. I am *not* advocating that a particular size or my specific weight is the "ideal" or should be *your* goals. I am attempting to share personal goals and how I accomplished them. Above all else, your goals should be in alignment with your "*why*" that you will determine in the following pages. Your health goals should be more than aesthetic and should include longevity and quality of life, more than the size of your jeans. So, let's just get *that* out of the way! In this book, I will help you to define and break through plateaus that you most likely will experience, as well.

Why Did I Write This?

I realize we are all different and there is no ONE magical fitness and nutrition plan for everyone. However, whatever you settle into, it should be maintainable as a lifestyle, not a short-term fix. When creating your goals, your priority should include increasing your overall health and increasing your ability to enjoy an active, vital lifestyle (free of debilitating health conditions) well into your 80's and 90's. I understand that we all have different aspirations — whether it is to look great in skinny jeans or keep up with our active children. However, if my research; my personal experiences; my mistakes and my victories can help you, then my hope is to guide you in every possible way. *Remember: health is a journey, not a destination. Therefore, choose to make it a joyful one!*

Now that you know *why* I wrote this book let's delve into the most important question you will need to ask yourself on your journey of health and wellness. In the next chapter, we will discuss the importance of finding your "why." **Don't skip this part.** It is crucial to your success! Of course, it is my desire that you achieve the *best* success possible.

Look your best. Live your best. Love your best.
All of the best to you,

Dr. Linné

Chapter 2
Find Your "Why"!
Getting Your Priorities Straight

Do Not Skip This!

Whatever you do, do *not* skip this part of your health journey. Too often we jump into the latest and greatest fitness or nutrition craze and inadvertently neglect the most important aspect of living a healthful lifestyle. As a result, negative consequences such as apathy, laziness —or even worse—giving up altogether, occur. Without a purpose for doing something; without a raison d'être, so to speak, our motivation for doing something new (and beneficial) is often lost in our daily tasks that may be less important, if significant at all. I'm guilty of it. We are all guilty of it, to some degree.

But if it is so important, then why do so many people forget this step before diving into a new nutrition or fitness plan? Well, if the answer was that simple, then I believe we would see many more fit, healthy individuals in this country. On the contrary, more than two-thirds of the U.S. population is either overweight or obese! And now, type 2 diabetes is showing up at astronomical rates in children! These types of health concerns were unheard of 50 years ago. We live in a day and age when convenience is king. We continually get bombarded with advertisements for food laden in highly processed forms of fat, sugar and unrecognizable ingredients. Therefore, it is no wonder we struggle so much as a nation to control our waistlines. And don't think for a moment that the food industry and the FDA, the organizations we look to for guidance on what is safe to eat, are more interested in the rising rate of heart disease and diabetes, than in making a profit. Yes, I just went there.

Why Should You Find Your "Why"?

So why do you need to know your *why* before you start this or any new beneficial lifestyle change? The reason is that motivation is key. Motivation is the key to creating and maintaining any fruitful and beneficial changes in your way of life. Think about a professional football team. Do you believe that the players would train hours a day, months on end, and play their hardest at every game if they played for free? Or, what if there were no playoffs and no Super Bowl? Would they play differently? What if their statistics were never tracked or kept on record? Would they work harder? Or would they want to give up after their first significant injury? You see for a football player motivation may be the money; the fame; the love of their team; the encouragement of their coach; the desire to go to the Super Bowl, etc. Motivation comes in many different forms; but, *without* motivation, there is *no* real reason to keep working toward a goal. For another example, how about a model? What motivates the model to stay in shape? Most likely he or she would lose their job if they gained weight or inches in the wrong places. Keeping their job may be motivation to eat right and to work out. Knowing that they may have to have their picture taken in scantily clad clothing on a moments notice, may be enough motivation to not overeat or drink at an event.

But, chances are you are not reading this because you are a professional football player or supermodel. Chances are, you are trying to find and identify what will motivate you to keep up the beneficial lifestyle changes that you are adopting and creating for yourself. So where do you start? Start by grabbing a piece of paper or your journal and brainstorm all of the possible reasons you may have for wanting to be healthier, fitter and in better shape. I recommend shying away from temporary motivators such as: "I want to look good at my sister's wedding" or " I want to look good for my trip to Mexico." While there is nothing wrong with these short-term goals, the motivation is not enough to keep you going after the wedding or after you return from your trip to Mexico.

Make It Count

Find motivators that are sustainable and relevant to you. For example, do you have active children that you want to be able to keep up with and play outside with; but, currently, you are too tired or too out of shape to do so? Do you have high cholesterol or blood pressure and you want to avoid all of the complications of heart disease or an early death? Do you want to have clearer thought processes because you are often unfocused and distracted? Do you want to sleep better because you often wake unrested? Do you want to try new sports but feel too out of shape? Do you want to be able to wear the size that will make you beam with pride when you put on those special pants? Do you want to reverse a disease process that has limited your optimism? Do you want more flexibility and obtain functional strength for daily tasks for as long as you are on this earth? Do you want to be able to travel, hike, bike and enjoy new places without feeling out of breath? Do you want to feel more confident in a bathing suit or naked?

Only you know what will motivate you as **your** *why. Write it down.* Then, when you get frustrated, or you feel like getting off track, you have something to come back to, a focus point. So, before starting a new nutrition or fitness program, write these things down, **now**! Keep them somewhere in your home where you can review them regularly — on your nightstand, the refrigerator, in a page of your journal, on your phone, etc. But, please, do NOT jump into any new health habit without first knowing *why* it is important to you.

Supercharge your health. Satisfy your soul. Simplify your lifestyle.

Write down your top three "Why" reasons, on a 3x5 card, NOW! Do not move on until you have completed this assignment. Once you have achieved this, then get ready! You are about to embark on the best-kept secret of weight loss: strengthening your mindset.

Chapter 3

Your Mindset Determines Your Success
Your Self Talk Matters

Reflect on Important People in Your Life

We have successfully determined the importance of finding your "why." You have your reasons in mind for why you are determined to adopt change. With your "why" clearly pictured, let's consider your closest friends and influencers in your life. Reflect on your life, and the times your friends, mentors, parents, teachers, pastors, etc. made you feel great about who you are and who you want to become. Do you have these people in mind? Now, think about their personality traits and characteristics. Were they positive when you were feeling cynical? Were they inspirational and upbeat? Did they always have the right thing to say when you needed a boost? Did they make you feel like you could conquer the world? Most likely, they made you feel great about who you are and what you have been created to do on this planet. Consequently, the more that these people encouraged you, the more you believed them — and as a result, you experienced great things come to fruition.

Now imagine with me, if you will, that you are approaching these same people with the frustrations you have about your health and your fitness level. Imagine if their response was something like:

> "You know you're never going to reach your goals, right? You've tried to get in shape before and look where that has got you! You're just going to give up. Your thighs are indeed fat, and your cellulite is disgusting! You need to cover that up and not think about buying a new outfit, today! If it looks bad in the dressing room, it won't look good out there! You're too old to get in good shape! Don't even think you'll be able to keep up with folks younger than you…"

Are You Your Worst Enemy?

These are offensive statements, aren't they? We can't even imagine people we admire and respect saying such things to us, can we? SO WHY ON EARTH DO WE SAY STUFF LIKE THIS TO OUR-SELVES…AND OFTEN? Our minds are amazing storage units for information. However, our minds cannot always determine true thoughts from untrue thoughts. Over time, given enough of the same thought patterns, the brain will develop a belief system sur-rounding similar thought patterns. More importantly, our habits (good and bad) will stem from these belief systems. And, conse-quently, our habits, over time, become who we are. This process of thoughts becoming beliefs and beliefs becoming habits is proven psychological science that I will not get into right now. However, many teachers and scientists demonstrate this to be the way our minds process the world around us. Our minds must have a method of categorizing the constant barrage of information we deal with day in and day out. By forming belief systems and maintaining habits, our mind can more easily make sense of all the information that filters through our brain. It is a method of categorizing, compartmentalizing and organizing information to create the world that we understand.

What's the Big Deal?

So what's the big deal? So what if you degrade yourself in the mirror or you have accepted your age limitations, and you own your genetic predispositions toward inheriting certain diseases? It's a fact of life, isn't it? Or, is it? On the contrary, if you tell yourself who you *want* to be or what you *want* to accomplish with *conviction*, in the *present* tense and *often*, expect *to* see dramatic changes in your current beliefs —and ultimately, expect to see changes in how quickly you accomplish your goals.

My weight loss journey, as aforementioned above, has been a long and fascinating journey. The journey has been an uphill battle at times, with plenty of plateaus along the way. While learning how to exercise properly *and* how to eat nutritionally sound food in proper proportions were important practices in breaking plateaus, it was not until I applied some critical mental activities, that I indeed saw a transformation take place. More important than the outward change was the internal transformation of my dialogue with myself, my beliefs surrounding my weight and my attitude toward an evolving lifestyle.

My Friend, Bob

In my journey, I met Bob, a friend, and my previous supervisor. Bob was responsible for pioneering the shift in my mental framework that allowed me to achieve success —the method that not only helped me create my ideal healthful body composition; but, discovering the ability to pursue and experience excellence in every other aspect of my life.

Bob introduced me to the concept of visualization and affirmations that he had learned from his mentors. Interested in becoming half as confident and determined as Bob, I started creating affirmations and a visualization practice, focused primarily on my health, in the beginning. Each morning I began my day with visualizing my ideal physique; the energy I wanted to feel; the act of putting on my favorite pair of jeans and smiling because I felt amazing, etc. I did this practice for 10 minutes. I also created a list of affirmations that supported the ideal picture I was visualizing. I recorded each of these affirmations on my phone with enough pause after each affirmation to repeat the statement. I practiced this ritual, daily, with feeling and conviction, in the car on my way to work.

This process was surprisingly refreshing and improved my mood and overall outlook by providing a sense of control and hope for my future. As time went by, I started to see the fruits of my thought patterns come to light; I began to see results. I felt more energetic than before. I started sleeping better. I was serendipitously coming across the right research; a good nutrition program; the appropriate exercise program at the right time. My mind was open and willing to accept the gifts available to me that would assist me in achieving my success. And all of this occurred with *little* effort on my part. Months later, I was able to achieve the goals I outlined in my affirmations to the exact pound, measurements, and body composition I desired.

Applying Your New Mindset

I have countless examples of how the gifts of affirmations and visualization have worked in my life. Not only have I completely changed my body, but I have also improved many of my relationships. I have passed excruciatingly difficult exams. I have completed projects that were seemingly impossible to complete...the list goes on and on. You see, the point is, that you *can* completely change the outcome of something —albeit, it may seem daunting at times. However, the feelings of doubt don't have to hold you back from improvement. Whether you wish to improve your weight or you want to alter your fears and your habits in other areas of your life, as you learn to change your mindset you can allow your subconscious mind to take over and do the driving, so to speak. Your improvements become automatic and require *minimal* effort on your part.

Getting Started With Your New Mindset

So where do you begin? You start by changing how you speak to yourself. And how do you do that? Grab a piece of paper (or your journal) and a pen and divide one page in half. Or, for this exercise, you can print off the Affirmation Worksheets from journeytowardjoy.com. You'll find these sheets under the Resources menu tab.

On one side, write down everything you dislike. Be specific. You may wish to start this process by addressing specific thoughts regarding your weight; your measurements; your physical performance; your flexibility; your energy level; your cholesterol level; your cellulite, etc. Once you have completed your "unhappy list," it is time to move over to the opposite page. Now, on the right side of the page write down your ideal characteristics that you wish to have—and again, be *specific*. Be specific to the pound, the inch, etc. For example, you may write on the left-hand side, "My thighs jiggle when I walk." On the right side of your paper, you may write, "Firm, slim, healthy, 22-inch thighs." Other examples of admirable qualities to include: Your ideal self can do 20 push-ups; you jump out of bed every morning refreshed and ready to start your day by 6 am, etc. Make your list as long as you wish. However, I cannot emphasize enough how important it is to be *very* specific. *The brain likes specifics!*

Now, here comes the fun part. You are going to create affirmations from your list on the right side. You can print off the Affirmation Worksheets from journeytowardjoy.com if a pre-made worksheet helps you. You'll find these sheets under the Resources menu tab.

These affirmations must be *positive*, in the *present* tense and *programmable*. What do I mean by programmable? Programmable is a term I use for affirmations that are simple enough for the brain to process and to adopt as a belief —and in turn, create subconscious habits to support this new belief.

To illustrate this process, I'll share with you some of my affirmations that I created for specific health-related areas I wanted to change. I should mention that of all of the affirmations I created; the *most important* statement to myself is: **"I love and accept myself unconditionally just the way I am."** I recommend you adopt this one, too. In fact, each time you catch yourself giving a returned look of disgust in the mirror, a negative thought creeps up in your mind, or you say something cruel to yourself, YOU NEED TO CORRECT YOURSELF BY SAYING THIS AFFIRMATION!!!

My Personal Favorites

Here are some of my specific affirmations for health and fitness:

- *"My skin is firm and smooth."*
- *"My body is dissolving excess fat for it no longer needs it."*
- *"I love how easy it is for me to maintain my excellent health, my set point of [X] pounds
  and my ideal body shape."*
- *"Each day, I feel more energetic and alive."*

- *"My nutritional intake supports my ideal health and body weight."*
- *"I am growing taller, more flexible, leaner and stronger every day."*
- *"I am a perfect size[X]."*
- *"I fall asleep quickly and remain asleep. Upon rising, my mind and body feel rested."*
- *"I get 7-8 hours of uninterrupted sleep every night."*
- *"Each morning I awaken feeling rested, energized and excited to start my day with purpose."*

Results You Can Expect

As a result of saying my affirmations, out loud, every morning, I have seen incredible results. I have surpassed the goals I set for myself—and as a result, I had to create new measurement and weight goals. I have grown to love and accept my body. For the first time in my life, I look forward to trying on clothes. So this process and method actually will work, *if* you make it work for you.

My Best Tips and Tricks

Also, I'd like to provide you with some essential tips and tricks to *crea*te an effective routine. Write every affirmation down concerning EVERYTHING you want. Make it *specific*. Make it *present tense* and make it **POSITIVE**. For example, do not say, "I'm not obsessed with eating bad foods." This type of statement has negative connotations. Instead, say, "I crave only the foods that nourish and fuel my body." I recommend recording yourself on your phone, saying each affirmation, and then pausing your voice for 5-10 seconds to allow enough time for repeating the affirmation, out loud, after each recorded statement. After all of the affirmations are recorded, you can now listen to your affirmations on a walk, jog or in the car and repeat them after hearing *your voice* say them. Hearing your voice is *very* powerful. If you don't want to record them, you can type them up and have them handy to read, out loud, as part of your morning routine.

When you repeat your affirmations out loud, say them with conviction and with emotion. Smile when you say them and say each of them like you are projecting on a stage. Say each one with power and with energy (a car is a perfect place for this, by the way). By adding emotion, you are further signaling the brain to make new neuronal connections to the belief you are creating. And, you will find that by adding the dramatized emotion, you may feel freakishly happier and excited for your day and what lies ahead.

Lastly, visualize yourself in shape; in the situation; in the form that you wish to create. Just as I benefited from imagining my ideal body and how it felt to be in it, you too will benefit from visualizing what it is that *you* want. Again, there is a lot of science behind the power of affirmations; but, I'll save that discussion for another time. However, feel free to research neurophysiology, neuroplasticity, cognitive psychotherapy and the power of affirmations, if you are interested.

After the process of addressing every aspect of your health that you wish to improve is complete, apply the same process to other aspects of your life. Use this process for your finances; your relationships; your spiritual walk; your business; your fears; your yearly goals; your intemperate habits, etc. Ultimately, every area of your life and every attitude you wish to change will benefit from creating new thoughts. I have *countless* examples of how the gifts of affirmations and visualization have worked in my life.

Getting to the Point

You see, the point is, that you *can* completely change the outcome of something. The feelings of doubt do not have to hold you back from improvement. Whether you wish to improve your weight or you want to alter your fears and your habits in other areas of your life, as you learn to change your mindset, you can allow your subconscious mind to take over and navigate you toward your goals. Your improvements become automatic and require *minimal* effort at all on your part. Remember, your thoughts become beliefs, which in turn, become your habits —and ultimately, become who you are. In other words: you are your thoughts.

Now it's your turn. What affirmations will you create around your ideal self? Make it fun! See the Affirmation Worksheets at journey-towardjoy.com to create lists and to create your affirmations.

TIP:

*Use the **Affirmation Worksheet A** located under Resources at <u>journeytowardjoy.com</u>. Use this resource to create lists, including the areas of your health that you wish to change and you are dissatisfied with, as well as a picture of your ideal. Include everything such as your weight; your measurements; your food choices; your blood pressure; your cholesterol; your hemoglobin a1C (if you know this number); your energy level; your strength and flexibility; your exercise choices, your stress levels, etc.*

*Once you have your list, it is time to create your affirmations from the "Ideal" column you created above, using **Affirmations Worksheet B** also located under the Resource tab at <u>journeytowardjoy.-com</u>. Make sure that your affirmations are in present tense, entirely positive and specific. If you need some assistance, I have added some examples for you here:*

"I quickly find ways to calm my mind and to create peace in my life."
"It is easy for me to create healthful boundaries with my time, my
relationships and my commitments."

"Every day in every way I am becoming leaner,
stronger, more flexible, and
more energetic."
"My doctors are shocked and amazed with my
glowing health reports."
"My hemoglobin A1C is below 5.5."
"Every day, I make choices in my food and activity
that lower blood
pressure and optimize my cholesterol levels."
"My Body Mass Index is in the preferred range of
18.5 to 24.9."
"I am feeling more and more energetic every day."
"I easily find time to exercise 5 times a week."

See it. Feel it. Believe it. Become it.

Before we dive into The Plan and how you are going to achieve optimum health, we need to discuss why some people gain weight so easily and can't get it off while others on the same plan get thin with little to no effort. In other words: you need to know that weight loss isn't just calories in and calories out! Do I have your attention? Yeah, I thought so.

Chapter 4

Weight Loss is About Calories and Activity, Right?

The Biggest Lie in the Diet Industry

Before we jump into the world of fat loss, it is important to understand that if you have struggled with weight loss; you have had the same pounds gained and lost over the years, despite eating relatively healthfully and participating in an active lifestyle, you are NOT alone. Just reducing calories and increasing exercise can lead to metabolic dysfunction. Metabolic dysfunction occurs when cutting calories (or carbohydrates for some) disrupts hormone balance. As a result of hormone disruption, the dieter can experience increased hunger, increased binge eating, decreased energy, a slower metabolism and a higher set point (the weight that the body prefers to be at). Each time one cuts too many calories to lose weight, this challenges the metabolism—and while there may be the monetary gain in a few pounds lost, it inevitably leads to the weight and fat coming back—and even more so—as the body fights back in a survival mechanism meant for storage. It never ends pretty when you fight your body's natural disposition toward survival.

I see this pattern of metabolic damage in nearly every patient coming to see me for weight loss. They are healthy, relatively active and have a history of either stress, a significant change of events (i.e., birthing a child, divorce, change in careers, etc.) or frequent dieting and exercise that has led to hormone resistance and the inability to burn fat. Even as a clinician and someone who researches the science behind weight loss and weight gain, I have fallen into the trap myself...Many times. Do you want to know the latest not-so-brilliant attempt at fat loss on my part? Of course you do! Everyone likes the dirty details, don't they?

As a woman, I am not impervious to the multitude of hormonal fluctuations and their effect on the body's tendency to store fat rather than burn it, if given the right circumstances. You have read my story at the beginning of this book and know that my weight loss journey has been an ongoing one as I strive toward challenging my body in beneficial ways and becoming the best version of myself.

Even as a type this, I am thinking of my most recent experimentation with a ketogenic diet, as it is the latest fad in our "dieting" culture. After much research, I decided to give the extremely low carbohydrate lifestyle a try. Feeling rather enthusiastic about how I initially felt; my increased energy; my symptom-free menses; my ability to fast regularly and the loss in water weight, I made a *fatal* dieting error. I let the enthusiasm take hold and decided to embrace the lifestyle wholeheartedly, without listening to other signs my body was giving me.

I fell into the trap of believing that if a little is helpful, then *a lot* is even better. You see, after observing the drop in water weight, I decided to make sure that my net carbohydrates (subtracting fiber from total carbohydrates) were under 50 grams every day. I embraced intermittent fasting with 24-hour fasts at least once a week and limiting my meals to two times per day. In my research, I discovered that the rate of metabolism is more dependent upon the total number of calories consumed in a day than the frequency of eating. Therefore, I deduced that if my caloric intake stayed the same, regardless of the frequency in which I ate, then getting all of my calories in two meals would only help my fat loss process, right? This method has worked for thousands of people who have tried intermittent fasting; therefore, it would certainly work for me!

Also, I applied the science of high-intensity interval training (HIIT), knowing that this type of exercise can increase fat burning up to 24-48 hours, post-workout. I stepped up my HIIT workouts to 20 minutes sessions, five days a week, knowing that I had "hit the holy grail of fat loss." After all, each of these tactics alone has been proven to burn fat. Combining all of these methods at once should be even better, right? To my dismay, I slowly started to see my hard-earned muscle definition slip away. The inches on every part of my body were slowly increasing. In a matter of months, I gained three inches on my hips and two inches on my waist, alone.

I was no longer able to feel powerful in my workouts and started to feel fatigued within 10 minutes. My strength suffered, and I went from easily completing 25 push-ups to barely finishing 5.

Despite the signs, I felt that I must stick with the program; that because the science supports the effectiveness of the diet and exercise methods, I must stick it out. I saw plenty of people online who achieved amazing results from the ketogenic diet so I determined that I must be patient and wait for the benefits to turn in my favor. I stuck to my guns for over two months. After testing my glucose one evening with my family, thinking I would win the award for the lowest and healthiest glucose levels in town, I was shocked to see that my levels were well above "ketogenic." What was going on? Why didn't I see favorable progress? Why wasn't my body changing for the better?

Determined to get to the bottom of the physiology behind my results (or lack thereof to say the least), I dug deep into the world of hormones, especially the body's hormonal responses to change in diet, exercise and fasting. What I discovered made so much sense that I knew I needed to alter my approach when helping others with their physical goals to lose weight. You see, our physique is not as much of a reflection of our caloric intake and our workouts as much as the hormonal shifts that take place on a day to day basis. Our food and our workouts can create hormone responses that can be favorable and unfavorable for fat loss. *Each person's hormonal makeup is as unique as their genetic makeup or their appearance.* Hormonal and genetic uniqueness vanquish any rationale that a "one size fits all" approach is *efficacious* in the diet industry. What works for one person, may not work for another as each has a unique hormonal makeup that provides an equally unique response to what one eats and how one moves the body.

So what happened in my case of hard-earned fat accumulation? In essence, the body responds to stress by releasing cortisol—which in turn, stimulates neuropeptide Y in the brain and other organs to increase fat storage. Also, high levels of cortisol can put the breaks on the thyroid and down-regulate the metabolism. Cortisol can increase the release of glucose into the blood stream; thus causing a spike in insulin which can lead to further fat storage. And, these are only a few of the effects that too much stress on the body will create. I was providing stressors in the form of too much intense activity, carbohydrate deprivation and dramatic changes in eating patterns (fasting). I was utilizing all three of these stressors to lose body fat, and it was backfiring.

Granted, lowering carbohydrates and occasional fasting can be *very* beneficial for many people. However, unless the person is metabolically sound and has a handle on their stress and adrenal health, then such changes can be deemed a stressor by the body—and thus, become a detriment to one's overall goals. Consequently, my adrenal health required rehabilitation after this experiment and I am much more careful when prescribing these methods to patients or friends and family. I achieved a slow progression toward recovery by limiting my HIIT workouts, increasing my yoga workouts, eating four to five meals per day and adding complex carbohydrates after my weight training or intense exercise. I stepped up my meditation and relaxation activities. Sure enough, the metabolic damage I created with my overzealous enthusiasm slowly started to reverse, given time, attention and a more intuitive approach.

What is the big take home, here? Metabolism is not about calories and exercise, as much as it is about hormone management. While reducing carbohydrates can be very beneficial for the body and improve overall health, for some folks, reducing carbs to zero can lead to increased cortisol levels, increase fat storage and a severely compromised metabolic function. I believe that if you have any history of stress, sleep dysfunction and cortisol imbalance, going very low-carb (below 50 net carbs per day) is not the right choice for you, at this time.

Now that you have read my experience with hormone misman-agement let's take a look at some of the players that are continually determining whether you will be burning fat or accumulating it. This list is not an extensive one by any means; but, you'll get an overall picture of how hormones and neurotransmitters work to-gether.

FAT-BURING HORMONES:

HUMAN GROWTH HORMONE

Human growth hormone (HGH) is a building and burning hor-mone. HGH signals body to be lean and muscular and works with adrenaline and cortisol to move in the direction of fat loss over fat storage.

THYROID

The thyroid gland is the body's fat burning engine. This tiny little tissue located in the middle of your neck impacts energy levels and acts as your body's thermostat. Like many glands in your body, it is susceptible to stress (and the stress of dieting) and the suppression induced by an overactive adrenal gland and an increase in stress (whether it is a pot of coffee, a fight with your spouse, traffic or extreme diet measures). For many folks, going too low in carbohydrates can negatively impact thyroid function. Interestingly enough, while the initial drop in carbohydrates causes insulin sensitivity, over time, the drop will cause an increase in cortisol levels and a decrease in leptin activity. The rise in cortisol and plummeting of leptin levels can lead to a release of glucose into the blood stream and increased hunger. Leptin acts directly on the thyroid, and low levels tell your thyroid to decrease energy output and to start storing fat. In turn, low thyroid levels will cause an increase in cortisol production, causing you to feel "wired, but tired." It is a vicious cycle. Thyroid hormone is disrupted by estrogen so that when estrogen is in excess, it can lead to a slower metabolism. The decrease in thyroid activity caused by estrogen dominance seems to be more true for women than for men, given women have higher levels of estrogen than men.

GHRELIN

Ghrelin is the hormone that impacts hunger and cravings. When ghrelin levels rise, this sends hunger signals to the brain. High ghrelin levels can be challenging to calm down with willpower alone. However, increasing water, fiber and protein can assist in suppressing the "gremlin" as I like to call it.

LEPTIN

Leptin is the new buzz word in the diet industry. Think of this hormone as the communicator between your fat storage and your brain. It tells your brain how much fat storage you have. Insulin resistance (insulin stops responding as readily to the influx of glucose), can be likened to leptin resistance in the brain (the brain stops listening to leptin). If the brain loses the ability to hear the signal (the consequence of chronic dieting) the brain produces leptin resistance and "ignores" the message. The result is dissatisfaction and continual hunger after a meal. Leptin manages thyroid hormone levels and thus can improve or disrupt the metabolic speed at which one burns fat.

INSULIN

Insulin is well-known and has been getting a rather bad rap in the diet community. However, insulin can be a friend, or it can be a foe. High levels of cortisol can lead to the storage of calories as fat. Insulin inhibits fat release. It makes fat cells very selfish and unwilling to let go of fat. However, insulin can also build muscle and control hunger. Having too much insulin leads to a softer body while having just the right amount, in response to an appropriate amount of carbohydrates, eaten at the right time, can lead to a firm, lean body.

INCRETINS:

Incretins include glucose-dependent insulinotropic peptide (GIP) and glucagon-like peptide (GLP). The small intestine produces glucagon-like peptides. The peptides sense the chemical composition of food. They tell the brain and pancreas (and other areas of the body) how to respond to the food that is coming. If the small intestines sense more sugar and fat is coming down the pipe, then more GIP is released. If more lean protein and vegetables are detected, then more GLP is released. Think of it like this: GIP is the "evil" fat-storing twin and GLP is the "good" fat-burning twin. Manage these two twins, and you can increase fat burning and weight loss by leaps and bounds.

STRESS HORMONES:

CORTISOL

Cortisol is our direct line to 911. It is the firefighter of the body. It has two sides to it much like insulin. The adrenals release cortisol with any perceived threat (fight with spouse, food allergy, intense exercise, caloric deprivation or carbohydrate deprivation, fasting, drinking a pot of coffee, traffic, a demanding boss at work, deadlines, etc.) During short bouts of stress (i.e., intense exercise), cortisol, adrenaline, HGH, and testosterone are released to *assist* in fat burning. When cortisol levels increase in the presence of elevated insulin, low testosterone and limited human growth hormone, it acts as a *fat-storing* and *muscle wasting* hormone. Increased corti-sol can also ramp up the reward centers of the brain (think dopamine depletion) and lead to sensations of cravings (i.e., the body seeks a dopaminergic response from a doughnut).

ADRENALINE:

Like cortisol, adrenaline lives in the adrenals (hence the name, of course). It is activated during a challenge and can signal fat burn-ing by turning on other fat-burning hormones (like HGH, testos-terone, cortisol, etc.). But, in the presence of high insulin and high leptin, it can cause cravings and lead to loss of muscle mass.

NEUROPEPTIDE Y:

Neuropeptide Y is a brain hormone that regulates hunger and is released by the nervous system when under chronic stress. It caus-es fat cells to amplify in number and size may be the reason that stress makes us fat. High levels of cortisol tell the nervous system to release more NPY and cause more fat storage. Here is my theo-ry: this may explain why initially, changes in carbohydrate intake, diet or exercise can have an immediate positive effect; but, if the changes are not beneficial long-term, then neuropeptide Y steps in and causes fat storage, despite the well-intentioned efforts. It all comes back to creating balance.

REPRODUCTIVE HORMONES:
DHEA

DHEA is the precursor to many hormones, including testosterone, estrogen, and progesterone. DHEA has been shown to be an indicator of overall health and longevity potential. There are many benefits to having higher levels of DHEA, including: the ability to keep cortisol in check; the decrease in "bad" cholesterol levels; make more thyroid hormone and the stimulation of libido (and testosterone formation). DHEA helps to convert thyroid hormone T4 into the active form, T3.

ESTROGEN/PROGESTERONE

There are cell receptors for estrogen and progesterone all over the body, including the brain, muscle and fat tissue. These sex hormones regulate reproduction but also affect fat burning and muscle building. Estrogen affects GABA, a neurotransmitter most known for its relaxing effect on the brain, as well as other neurotransmitters such as serotonin, and dopamine. The right amount of estrogen can help maintain thinness; but, an increase in estrogen leads to fat storage in the hips, butt, and thighs. The right amount of estrogen sensitizes the body to insulin and blocks the negative effects of cortisol, making it easier to tolerate stress and shape muscle, while storing less fat. Progesterone works as estrogen's counterpart and makes women more likely to store fat and liable to lose muscle. When levels of progesterone drop, this can lead to moodiness, hunger, and cravings. Progesterone also collaborates with estrogen to block cortisol.

TESTOSTERONE

This hormone in both men and women helps to shape and build muscle. Also, adequate levels of testosterone can improve almost every aspect of well-being including your assertiveness, motivation, energy levels, mental health, cognition and memory, bone strength and heart health, improved appearance of skin, etc. Too much testosterone can lead to polycystic ovary syndrome (PCOS) in women.

NEUROTRANSMITTERS:

Think of neurotransmitters as the switches that can turn on or turn off other hormones in the body. Neurotransmitters act as the fuse box, and the hormones are the light bulbs. If you don't have enough power in the fuse box, your lights won't turn on. In a perfect world, the stimulatory and inhibitory neurotransmitters are in balance, and the nervous system is excited when necessary and then buffers the stimulation swiftly and efficiently once the short-term stressor has passed. Neurotransmitters control all communication that occurs throughout your brain and body. Ultimately, the action of every organ, tissue, and cell rely on neurotransmitters for communication that will turn on or turn off activity of hormones. Quite often an imbalance of hormones is tied directly to an imbalance of the stimulatory or inhibitory neurotransmitters. Thus, the issues of weight gain and fat loss resistance must be viewed in light of the nervous system's relationship to—and governance of, the endocrine and immune system to fully understand how to "fix" the problem.

In the nervous system, the neuronal cells do not touch each other; but, rely on neurotransmitters to send signals to the target site cell receptors. Once the message arrives, a cascade of physiological actions helps to regulate such things as emotion (fear, pleasure, joy, sadness, etc.), concentration, alertness, energy, appetite, cravings, sleep, pain, etc. When balanced, the nervous system provides a proper checks and balances system to maintain homeostasis at all times. Concerning weight management, an imbalance of neuro-transmitters can lead to obesity, insulin resistance, food addictions, compulsive eating, slow metabolism, etc. Let's take a look at each neurotransmitter and how they each relate to your health and well-being.

GABA

GABA is one of two inhibitory neurotransmitters. It is a calming chemical. In fact, it acts as a very effective sedative and helps neu-rons recover after a bout of excitatory action. Think of it as the friend who can calm you down after someone ticked you off. When it is low, this can lead to anxiety, a lack of stress resilience, irritability and impulsive behavior. Too high levels are usually a result of the excitatory neurotransmitters being out of balance— and thus, acting as a compensatory mechanism.

SEROTONIN

Serotonin is the other inhibitory neurotransmitter switch. While we often associate low levels serotonin with depression and mood dis-orders, serotonin is also intimately related to digestion and appetite. Also, serotonin is the precursor to melatonin production in the pineal gland—and thus, plays a significant role in sleep patterns. When it is too high, stress resilience goes down; sleep suffers, inflammation rises and poor nutrition ensues. Too low levels of serotonin cause depression, compulsive behaviors, increased carbohydrate cravings, PMS, decreased pain tolerance and sleep disturbances. Regarding weight issues, serotonin determines one's level of motivation. Depletion of serotonin may result in the lack of impulse control, and the inclination to satisfy cravings goes up. As a result, an individual will crave starches and sugars to mimic serotonin in the brain when levels are imbalanced. The ideal, or "the Goldilocks range" as I call it, causes feelings of self-worth, happiness, and satisfaction in life. The pot is sweetened when these pleasant feelings come wrapped up in a lovely box of proper stress adaptation and restful sleep at night.

DOPAMINE

Dopamine can function as both excitatory and inhibitory, depending on which site on a cell it attaches. Dopamine regulates the reward and pleasure-seeking centers of the brain and thus plays an active role in addiction. Also, dopamine can assist with memory, motor skills, motivation, and interest. When it is low, there is little motivation to complete tasks, energy is low, and there is often a lack of concentration. Low dopamine can cause folks to self-medicate with drugs—or in respect to weight—with food. Issues with dopamine and PEA lead to either overeating or under eating. The pleasure reward pathway is driving this. If these two neurotransmitters are deficient, you will seek food for a reward.

NOREPINEPHRINE

Norepinephrine (also called noradrenaline) boosts function of your brain and is a fit-or-flight response and survival mechanism to help assess danger and gauge opportunity for survival. Too much of this chemical causes anxiousness and hyperactivity. Too low levels can cause apathetic behavior, fatigue, lack of motivation and foggy brain. Norepinephrine is involved in T4 to T3 conversion in the thyroid. If you can't do this conversion, the thyroid becomes sluggish, and the metabolism slows down. Just the right amount of norepinephrine—or the Goldilocks range, combats stress, inflammation and improves sleep and concentration.

EPINEPHRINE

Epinephrine (or adrenaline) is essential to metabolism. It regulates arousal and attention and inhibits insulin, releasing fatty acids into the blood stream. Low levels result in fatigue, difficulty focusing and trouble losing weight. High concentrations cause insomnia, anxiety and the inability to focus. The adrenals release both norepinephrine and epinephrine in times of stress. Short term this is beneficial. However, long term stimulation can lead to adrenal dysfunction. Neurotransmitters and their effect on insulin and glucose are relatively clear-cut relationships. In fact, norepinephrine and epinephrine govern feeding and regulate insulin and glucose. Too much norepinephrine causes the hypothalamus to overproduce cortisol in the adrenals. Unfortunately, stress drains serotonin stores, breaking the calming mechanism. With an increase in stress and inflammation, the body increases its need for a serotonin-like calming affect—and because excessive stress has depleted sero-tonin stores— you feel the need to eat a lot of sugar to mimic the effects of serotonin on the nervous system. It is a vicious cycle of stressors, inflammation and compensatory eating habits which cause more stress and more inflammation, perpetuating a down-ward spiral of weight gain. The inflammatory cycle leads to insulin resistance as well as leptin resistance making matters worse.

GLUTAMATE

Glutamate is the major player in creating excitatory action in the brain. Low levels create fatigue and decreased brain activity. High levels can contribute to many clinical neurological diseases, in-cluding depression, OCD and much more. In the Goldilocks range, glutamate assists in learning and memory. Glutamate reinforces associations between environment and behavior. When glutamate is higher than dopamine, you have trouble with impulse control. It becomes tough to resist tempting foods. Environmental cues will be too much for the person. For example, imagine walking near a doughnut shop and not being able to pass by it. You have to buy a dozen and eat them all. The recurring cycle of poor self-control occurs when glutamate is high, and dopamine is low.

HISTAMINE

Histamine is commonly involved in immune reactions but rarely is histamine associated with its other actions that affect emotions and behavior. Low histamine contributes to low libido, fatigue, sensi-tivities, etc. High levels lead to compulsive behavior, depression, and headaches. The Goldilocks range assists in regular sleep-wake cycles and promotes the proper release of epinephrine and nor-epinephrine.

PEA

PEA (or phenylethylamine) is an excitatory neurotransmitter, made from the amino acid phenylalanine. When it is high, it causes mind racing, sleep problems, anxiety, etc. When it is low, PEA is associated with difficulty paying attention and with depression. However, the Goldilocks range allows for proper focus and concentration. An interesting fact is that PEA (from phenylalanine) and serotonin (from tryptophan) directly stimulate the gut to produce a hormone called Cholecystokinin (CCK). CCK provides appetite control (satiation) and stimulates the pancreas to produce enzymes and insulin; stimulates the gallbladder to squirt bile into gut and CCK shuts down the hunger signals in the brain to create satiation.

ENZYME ACTIVITY RELATED TO FAT LOSS:

There are several gatekeepers on the cell membrane that determine if fat will be stored or released. Lipoprotein lipase (LPL) is the enzyme that lets fat "in the door" and acts to store fat. Think of him as a doorman who lets fat into the cell. His counterpart, hormone-sensitive lipase (HSL), is the doorman who opens the door to release fat. The boss of lipoprotein lipase is insulin. Insulin tells LPL to let fat into the cell. Adrenalin, the boss of hormone-sensitive lipase, orders HSL to release fat. Adrenaline has two choices of doors to use when releasing fat. The options for fat-releasing doors are alpha receptors and beta receptors. Alpha receptors allow a trickle of fat to be released (think of a revolving door that only allows one to two people leave at a time). Beta receptors allow a flood of fat to be released (think garage door at a Costco). Stubborn fat areas (i.e., back of arms, stomach, but, hips and thighs) have more alpha receptors and therefore release fat much more slowly. Whereas, the areas of the body that are rich in beta receptors will lose fat more quickly.

In addition to insulin, estrogen enhances the activity and number of alpha adrenergic receptors. And, in addition to adrenaline, thyroid hormone increases beta receptor activity and blocks alpha receptors. However, thyroid is controlled by estrogen and adrenal activity so that when these two are elevated, thyroid activity diminishes. Another interesting fact is that there is less blood flow in alpha adrenergic receptor dense areas.

SUMMARY

If all of this sounds like the makings of a juicy soap opera, then you are correct. All of these chemical messengers are intertwined and reactive with one another. At any given time, all of these chemical agents are at play. Whether or not the body burns fat or stores fat, is solely dependent upon which hormones are activated and which ones are buffered. In other words: fat loss cannot be simply a matter of how many calories you eat in a day or if you exercise.

Does the discussion of hormone fluctuation in the body seem likened to a crazy episode of "As The Body Fat Burns" (I thought of that soap opera title, myself [insert an eye roll, here])? It is clear that hormone and neurotransmitter fluctuation determine whether the body will lose or gain weight. Additionally, hormones and neurotransmitter determine one's ability to break a plateau, curb cravings and hunger, avoid fatigue after a meal, etc. We must stop believing the lie that weight loss is only about how many calories you consume and how active you are. Every—and I mean every—patient that I work with has had an issue with hormone function that contributes to a slower metabolism and higher than desired set point. None of my patients are couch potatoes that stuff their face with cartons of ice cream and potato chips every night. While their diet may need a few tweaks here and there, over consumption is usually not the issue. It is almost always related to an imbalance in stimulation of the hormones that store fat or suppression of those needed to burn fat. In most folks struggling with weight, it is a combination of both scenarios, thus creating the perfect storm for fat accumulation.

So what is the answer to sustained fat loss? How do you "train" hormones to behave in the manner you prefer? Can hormones even be trained? This question is a reasonable and yet it requires a rather complicated answer. While it warrants an extensive response, the simple answer is "yes." Hormones can be trained through proper nutrition, provided at the right intervals, under the right circumstances and in combination with the right types of exercise and appropriate lifestyle changes.

The answer begins with starting with the basics. In the next couple of chapters, I'll help break down the mystery of food and provide a list of foods for you to begin your journey. You will learn how to eat, how often and how much to turn on your metabolism. You will also learn how to listen to your body to know what adjustments you should make in your macronutrients (protein, carbohydrates, and fat) to maintain your weight or continue to lose fat. Also, You will learn what exercises will burn the most fat and how often you should engage in these activities. And, as with food, you will learn how to make the necessary adjustments to your exercise routine to keep the flame burning. The food lists I have chosen are specifically designed to provide your body with the proper fuel for balance, support, and vitality.

I will walk you through each detail that will help you to determine the best place to start *for you*. Each person has a different starting point, and each has a different chemical makeup. Once you get these two lifestyle adjustments under control (nutrition and exercise), you can make further adjustments and tailor your plan to either forge more fat loss or to maintain your progress. I'll teach you exactly how to make these changes, in a simple formulated manner. Don't worry.

If your head is spinning with all of the details, just know that this book is not meant to be the cookie cutter method that applies to everyone. Instead, it is intended to empower the reader to understand the cues and clues to look for when aspiring to create optimal change in health and vitality. This book provides you with the steps necessary to make adjustments, one new change at a time. I cannot emphasize the importance of ONE change at a time and give each change a minimum of one to two weeks for the body to catch up and respond. By paying attention to your body and how it responds to change; by tracking your response to food and exercise, you will have all the tools you need to create the desired hormonal response required to create the body that you want.

You now understand mindset and the importance of making sure you have your "why" before you start any program—be it this one or another. You understand that weight loss is a complex intertwining of chemicals in the body more than it is about how much food you eat and how often you exercise. In the next chapter, before we discuss nutrition, we need to make sure that you are fully prepared to be successful. Before starting any diet and exercise program, it is necessary to establish groundwork that will safeguard your success. Without this groundwork, you are less likely to maintain your momentum toward greatness and to the lifestyle you desire. But, you are motivated and ready, aren't you?

Chapter 5
Preparing for Success

Get Your House in Order!

For some of you, this will be the most difficult part of the process and journey toward an optimum healthful lifestyle: getting started by letting go. However, if you want to succeed at becoming the best version of yourself and achieve ultimate health and wellness, you are going to have to determine what is more costly to you. Will you choose the cost of the food you need to toss or the cost of your future medication that you have to purchase monthly for the rest of your life! Yes, it is money you are tossing away when you throw out "perfectly good food"; however, if the food item is *not* contributing to your overall fitness and health, then it is *sabotaging* your fitness and health. You need to make a choice. Will it be $150 in groceries that you toss and give away today or will it be $150 in medications every month in your future? Have you made your decision yet? If you can't toss it out, then please don't bother moving on to the next steps because you are not at the point where it is important enough, yet. Your health has to be more important than the original decision you made to buy the processed food because it "sounded good." Your health has to be more important than the cost of the bag of Doritos. And trust me, once you toss out such items, you will be more careful about your future purchasing decisions. As an added benefit, it is more likely that you will be utilizing everything you buy because you will be making *smart* purchasing choices in the future.

So, your first step is to take an hour or two and go through every cupboard and every shelf of your kitchen and pantry. Toss everything that has added sugar, hydrogenated fat, corn syrup, ingredients you cannot pronounce, etc. Throw out all nut butter with hydrogenated oil, salad dressings, and sauces lacking whole food ingredients (you should make your own, anyway), sugary snacks (except dark chocolate on the approved list), chips, crackers, cookies, bread, buns, and rolls. If it is not on the approved list, or contain ingredients from the approved list, then toss it!

You will *not* thrive with this program if you continue to fuel your body with canola, corn, soybean, and cottonseed oils. Nor will you thrive with any chemical-laden sweeteners (aspartame, saccharin, Splenda, Sucralose). You certainly will not succeed if you continue to spike your insulin levels with heavy carbohydrate meals throughout the day; thus, preventing you from being in a fat burning state. So, get rid of anything that has sugar as an ingredient (you'll be shocked how many condiments, dressings, boxed foods, and canned or jarred foods have sugar). Get a buddy to help you, if you are having separation anxiety from your corn chips. YOU. CAN. DO. THIS. Don't worry; you won't be craving these things anyway in a few days—especially after you see the scale numbers and your measurements, move in the right direction.

The most obvious method of preparation, as aforementioned above, is drastically clearing out your home of all temptation and processed junk. It clutters your refrigerator and cabinets as well as your body. You cannot get serious about making a change without letting go of food clutter. It is that simple. Again, get someone to help you if you need.

Once you clean house, you are ready to start the program.

> *As a bonus, you will save money in the long run because you will not be buying processed juices, sauces, and foods that you can make yourself at a lower cost.*

Food Preparation is Key

In a couple of chapters, I will introduce you to "The Plan." As part of your preparation, I will provide you with an extensive list of Approved Foods. You will need to find time to grocery shop and prepare some food ahead of time to assist you with your success. I find that one of the biggest reasons that people make poor food choices is because they have not stocked up on healthful choices or they haven't properly planned or prepared in advance. Always bring some snacks and drinking plenty of water, when leaving the house.

Before you begin this eating plan, I suggest you find some recipes that follow the guidelines in this book (or use the ones I have provided) and determine what meals you wish to have for the following week. Once you have decided what you want to eat for the week, make a list of any food items that you will need to pick up and get your home properly stocked. Additionally, if you want to earn some extra credit and sanity, you can cook items in bulk on a weekend day and have them available throughout the week. You can cut up your fresh veggie snacks or cook some of my meal recipes. Why not cook a large batch for the week? Roast a bag full of broccoli, cauliflower, etc. Cook a dozen hard boiled eggs. You can barbecue some steak, fish or chicken if you wish and have some handy. Make homemade dressings, BBQ sauce, mayo, etc. so you have some to grab something quickly when you are on-the-go. As part of preparing ahead of time, I find that picking one day on the weekend to prepare foods for the week, ensures that I am successful.

Even if you don't want to cook in bulk, you should always prepare to have snacks handy in your car or purse whenever you leave the house. You should also have a quart of water with you. Otherwise, you will be pulling into the nearest taco bell—and before you know it—you'll be wondering why there is a cheese burrito in your hand and why you are feeling ill shortly after its consumption.

Get the Right Tools

In addition to having the right foods in your home, please consider having the right utensils and appliances to make your life easier. While none of these are necessary, they certainly make life easier.

Here are just a few of my favorite kitchen tools that I use almost on a daily basis:

TIP:

Make sure you check out the Resource menu at journeytowardjoy.com to find the shopping list that I use when grocery shopping for all of my ingredients.

- **Powerful blender** (I like KitchenAid); but, a Vitamix is great, too!
- **Slow cooker** (I use my **Instant Pot** every day, and it can cook poultry meat in less than 20 minutes)
- **Food processor** (this comes in handy when making dressings, pesto, etc.)
- **Stainless steel pots and pans** (avoid non-stick cookware as these can release toxins into your food).
- **Juicer** (I like my Breville; but, you may want to consider a high-quality slow juicer that allows you to get the most of your fruits and vegetables, such as Omega 8006).
- **Citrus juicer**
- **Water heater** (I LOVE our Cuisinart temp-controlled water heater that allows us to choose the temperature based upon our beverage choice).
- **Parchment paper** this has helped to create pizza crust and other baking dishes with a no mess and no hassle clean up.
- **A good knife set** You don't need a lot of cooking knives. In fact, two great ones will cut most anything.

- **Spirilizer** (a.k.a zucchini noodle maker)

Drink a Minimum of Half of Your Body Weight, in Ounces, of Water!

Ideally, drink your body weight in ounces of water. A quart of water is 32 oz, so, for example, if you weigh 150 pounds, you will drink approximately 4 quarts of water per day. Sounds like a lot? Yes, it is; however, it will keep you satiated, hydrated, detoxified, will assist in fat removal from the body and will decrease inflammation and bloating. I suggest you drink the first quart within 20 minutes of waking.

Allow Yourself Regular Cheats of Chocolate or Wine!

This plan is supposed to be rewarding, satisfying and move you toward a lifestyle you can maintain, *without* the pain. Find recipes that utilize the approved foods and explore some options of your own.

However, as you are starting out, keep a **Meal and Serving Tracker** (found at journeytowardjoy.com under the menu item listed as Resources) on your refrigerator to make sure that you are getting all of the nutrients your body needs and to avoid overeating. Tracking your servings is key to your success. It wasn't until I started tracking my portions that I noticed the weight finally started to come off. I wasn't paying attention to how much protein, fat, and carbohydrates I was getting and couldn't figure out why my weight wouldn't budge. Even with counting calories, it is important to keep your macronutrients (protein, fat, and carbohydrates) relatively in check. You can do this, simply by tracking your number of servings.

Limit The Foods in the Approved List Labeled as Such (*)!

If your intent is to decrease inflammation in the body and insulin resistance, it is best to move toward as much of a grain-free, dairy-free, legume-free, sugar and alcohol-free diet as possible. However, because this diet is not meant to deprive you, there are limited, approved amounts of these foods that are acceptable, if you just can't help yourself. Please be aware that if you notice that your weight will not budge, these items may be contributing to a frustrating plateau.

Sleep!

Getting enough rest is essential for fat loss, hormone balance, immune-boosting, detoxification and mental rebooting. You cannot achieve the optimum in these areas without adequate sleep hygiene. What tips and tricks do I have up my sleeve that you can start utilizing now to improve your sleep hygiene?

Head to bed at 10 pm.

Research demonstrates that every hour you sleep before 12 am is worth two hours of quality sleep. If you think you are a night owl, you are not. You have just trained yourself to be one, or you have a neurotransmitter or hormonal imbalance (or both) that you can address with proper testing and supplementation. However most, people can benefit from going to bed 1/2 hour earlier for a week, then another 1/2 hour earlier the following week until you are in bed by 10 pm.

Use blackout shades or an eye mask.

You can purchase solid blackout fabric at your local fabric store and cut the right size for your bedroom windows if you don't need something fancier. Otherwise, the investment in beneficial blackout shades is well worth the outcome.

Turn your phone on airplane mode and place it more than 4 feet away from your bedside.

If you have been living in a cave, then you may not know that your phone enables Wi-fi and allows for radio-frequency electromagnetic fields to be present near your body. While studies remain inconclusive as to whether or not cell phone emissions cause brain cancer, it is common knowledge that your brain is an electrical jungle that needs as little disruption as possible in an effort to repair and process information during the night. Many people report less interrupted sleep when their phone is on airplane mode and away from their bedside. Also, the light from your phone (if checking emails, browsing the web, etc. before bed) can inhibit the production of melatonin in the pineal gland—and as a result, will hamper the sleeping process.

Have a pre-bed ritual.
My favorite routine looks something like this:

> A) Take the time to read a book with a calming cup of valerian or chamomile tea.

> B) Take a hot, candlelit bath (add Epsom salts and a few drops of lavender) while listening to jazz music. The magnesium in the Epsom salts is perfect for relaxing muscles and detoxifying your system (add in a glass of dry red wine, if you wish. Just don't have more than one glass as alcohol may disrupt your sleep patterns).

> C) Do some light yoga stretching now that your muscles are warm.

> D) In a journal beside your bed, write down the three things you wish to accomplish the next day that move you closer toward your goals. I like to add: "What did I learned about myself, others and the world, today?" "What did I accomplish today?" and "What am I grateful for?" The answers to these questions can provide a beneficial outlook on life, necessary for reflection. By assessing your daily

life, you become more present and more aware of small achievements and observations. Also, journaling provides the opportunity to ask questions to which you seek answers. Write your questions down and let your mind process them through the night. Keeping a journal beside your bed also helps with those "aha" moments in the middle of the night.

E) Finish with a nighttime meditation from your favorite YouTube channel or phone application (see **Appendix** for starters). I suggest one that focuses on stress and anxiety, gratitude or forgiveness. I also like following a guided meditation that helps me to visualize my ideal day, in preparation for the next day. My current favorite is "The Six Phase Meditation" found on YouTube.

Of course, you can create your own routine. The purpose is to have a method for calming your body and mind down; rather than, stay up watching television, working on your computer or responding to Facebook feeds and texts on your phone.

Avoid blue light (from T.V., computer, and phone screens) one to two hours before your scheduled bedtime.
By avoiding electronics, your body produces more melatonin and aids in improving sleep patterns. Having a routine that eases you into sleep can be very beneficial to your mind, body, and soul. You can use the computer program "f.lux" to adjust the display color of

your PC or digital device and filter out light patterns that strain eye and disrupt sleep patterns. You can also program your devices to be in night-time mode, if the option in your system preferences for display options, is available. If you must partake in electronic interaction before bed, you can also try getting orange glasses to block the blue light from your electronics. However, proper sleep hygiene preferentially includes turning off your electronic devices an hour or two before bedtime.

Consider using white noise with an air purifier.
An air purifier will help to keep the air clean that you breathe while you sleep and assist in drowning out any outside noises (think birds in the morning, trains, traffic noise, etc.). You can also download an application on your phone for white noise. Just make sure your phone is on airplane mode and away from your bed. Some folks like the app "brain FM" to assist in brain entrainment that enables focus/creativity/sleep. With this phone app, you are encouraged to wear headphones while you sleep.

Use an oil diffuser with comforting aromas.
Choose from a variety including bergamot, cedar, clary sage (my favorite), coriander, frankincense, lavender, Roman chamomile, sandalwood, sweet marjoram (another favorite) and ylang ylang. Feel free to mix and match these to create your ideal blend

Ditch the caffeine after 12 pm.

It goes without saying that too much of a stimulant can prevent your body from sleeping. Your liver needs plenty of time to detoxify stimulants from your system before bedtime. So, help your liver out and get your fix in the morning if you must.

Avoid eating three hours before your scheduled bedtime.
The majority of fat burning, rejuvenation, cellular turnover, and brain rebooting takes place while you are sleeping. If your body is busy metabolizing food, you lose out on these benefits to some extent. Why would you want to cheat your body of burning off some extra fat or clearing away mental cobwebs and stress?

Exercise daily and in the morning.
There are plenty of studies that support exercise and the quality of sleep. Keep in mind that working out before bed may amp up your energy levels; and therefore, sabotage your pre-bed calming efforts.

Keep temperatures cool in your bedroom.
Studies show that a temperature between 60 and 65 degrees Fahrenheit will modulate body temperatures better while you are sleeping. Better body temperature means better circadian rhythm and more sound sleep patterns.

Tips for eating out

It is important to plan and prepare before eating out. Determine how many servings of each food group you have eaten that day and to research the restaurant menu, online, to see if healthy options are available to you. Call ahead and ask if food preparation can be altered to meet your needs.

When ordering meat, fish or poultry, ask to have it grilled with a non-vegetable oil and request more healthy options (olive oil, avocado, coconut, sesame, etc.). Avoid fried, breaded foods. Pass on any potatoes, pasta or starchy dishes and opt for steamed or grilled vegetables instead. When ordering a salad, omit the croutons, tortilla chips, beans, corn, and cheese. Ask for the dressing on the side and eyeball about two tablespoons in your application. Vinaigrettes are usually the safest bet. Always pass on the bread bowl or chips and salsa and let your waitress know ahead of time as a courtesy.

If you need a munchie before you food arrives, order a grilled vegetable appetizer, a shellfish (i.e., muscles) or any other allowed food on the Allowed Foods list. Save a glass of wine for after your meal in place of a desert. Or, you can have a cup of coffee. Make sure you load up on water before dining out and fill up on a fibrous snack so that you are not famished when you arrive at the restaurant and start attacking the bread bowl.

When Attending Special Events, Dinners, and Parties

Again, it is important to prepare yourself mentally *before* you arrive at any party. Think about your progress and what you have accomplished. Have you lost weight? Is your digestion better? Do you feel less bloated? Do you have more energy? Do your joints hurt less? Also, always have your *"why"* in mind. You have chosen to make this enormous step toward ultimate health and fitness for a reason, and this reason must always be at the forefront of your mind so that when you are offered birthday cake at the next party, you may respond appropriately.

You may be thinking to yourself, "But what if I offend my friends and family by turning down their homemade devil's food cake?" This question is a valid one. Think about it from a new perspective. Do friends and family care about you and your health? They should! Do your closest friends and relatives know your intention to become the healthiest version of yourself? They should! It is important to make this known to them *before the invitation to a party.*

When the time comes for you to attend the party or dinner, have the food choices that you *can* have, in mind. Know how many servings of each food category you have left for the day and how many cheats you can have and save some room for the event you are attending. You do not need to have a little bit of everything served because "someone made it with love." If they care about you and your health, they will know why you are working toward staying on track and will support you in your efforts.

What to do With "Food Pushers"

There will be the food pushers in your life that say things such as, "Oh come on! A little cake isn't going to hurt you!" You will need to prepare by formulating a response ahead of time. For example, if your *"why"* is to decrease inflammation in your body, and improve your blood glucose levels, you may respond by saying, "Thank you for your offer. The cake looks incredible; however, if I am going to enjoy many more parties in my future, I need to stay on track with my health and my choices, now." Or, you can try, "Thank you for the kind gesture. Your food looks like it belongs in a magazine! However, when I eat [x] I don't feel as vital the next day, so I am going to have to pass."

Before you attend an event, make sure your mental focus is on how you will feel later after having food that isn't a "vitality promoter" and focus on *why* you have chosen to eat clean. Think about how you will feel an hour after you eat the cake or how you may feel for the rest of the week. Ask yourself how you got to be overweight, have high blood pressure, have sore joints, feel lethargic or less focused, in the first place. Did it happen overnight? No! Your health conditions or your weight occurred slowly, over time, one food choice at a time. Likewise, your turnaround will only happen *one food choice at a time*. With this in mind, ask yourself, "Is this one dinner; this one party; this one meal worth the risk of derailing me from my momentum? Is this piece of cake worth feeling bloated afterward and noting that my scale has gone up a bit in the morning? Is it worth having sore joints tomorrow?" I'll leave the answer to these questions up to you. But, trust me, if you are serious about your health, you will find ways to say "no" to the "food pushers" in your life. When you are serious about your goals, there is *no piece of cake will ever amount to the way you feel when your health is on track or when you no longer have to sausage squeeze yourself into your pants!!*

What if I Cheat or "Get Off Track"?

Now, does preparing for parties and standing up to Food Pushers mean you should torture yourself and never have the foods you love? Well, there are several ways for me to answer that. The natural progression of optimum nutrition will eventually lead you to a loss of cravings, overall. You will crave less sugar over time. Foods that once brought you "joy" may start to bring you pain as you become more in tune to your body. In other words: you will start to prefer the way vegetables make you feel over a pop tart. In fact, you will feel a bit sick when you think about eating any processed food. The newfound aversion is a natural consequence of choosing to clean up eating habits.

If you haven't picked up on it already, you should know that this diet plan is not about depriving yourself. You are allowed your daily cheats, in moderation, if you choose to have them. However, every once and a while you may want to have a sweet dessert. That's fine! Plan for these days, so you are not unprepared. I know I say this a lot, but *preparation is your key to success!*

Plan on having that fancy desert, *every once and a while*; but NOT regularly, and make sure you track your calories that day so that you factor the "fun" food into your caloric requirements. Think of it as a food budget. If you know you want to have a 500 calorie piece of pie, and your "budget" provides 1,300 to 1,500 calories of food, then you know you can "spend" 1,000 calories of food in addition to your "fun" food. But, here's the catch: opt for foods that reasonably follow your plan. For example, a flourless chocolate cake or pumpkin pie *without* the crust and whip cream. Avoid the foods that will cause you pain or inflammation (i.e., grains, dairy, allergens, too much sugar, etc.).

Make sure the serving size is reasonable and *don't opt for seconds!* Another tip is to opt for a fruit bowl with homemade chocolate syrup. You don't need the shortcake with your bowl full of strawberries. Instead, add a dollop of whip cream, and voila! You have a treat that won't break your calorie "bank." And, most importantly, make your occasional "fun" WORTH IT!!! Make sure it is decadent and something you love, not a processed boxed treat that you feel guilted into trying. Eat it very slowly and ENJOY it! You don't want guilt associated with something that is ok to do every once and a while. That is why planning is so important, so you know what to expect, and you can enjoy the food without the guilt. Trust me. You will thank me the next day. Trust me.

It also helps to eat something fibrous to fill you up (i.e., apple, a Keto Coffee or my smoothie recipe), before attending a party or gathering. You don't want to stand near the hors d'oeuvres table on an empty stomach. Also, drink all of your body weight in ounces of water on the days you are attending an event to keep you full, satisfied and hydrated.

Now, what do you do if you fell off the wagon and are desperate for a reboot? Follow the bonus tips below for an easy, non-painful way to get refocused. But, whatever you do, please do not continue to eat the same way, the next day. Get back on your horse and continue back on the path toward your optimum health. Whatever you do, DON'T BEAT YOURSELF UP! We are all human and will make choices we regret from time to time; but, we always have the ability to turn it around and make tomorrow a better day.

Simple Solutions for Quick Weight Loss (If You Need to Get Back on Track or You are Preparing for a Special Event)

At any time during your weight loss journey, you may feel your body needs a reboot. Whether you have "fallen off of the wagon" or you want to do a simple detox, you can come back to this section of the book and get yourself back on track toward success. Consider this your fail safe method for "righting" any "wrongs," should you need a quick fast-track getting back on your optimum health path.

For one to three weeks, eliminate both servings of complex carbohydrates, if you have not already done so. Drink your body weight in ounces of water per day. Drinking this much water will be challenging so feel free to use the water recipes provided in the **Recipes** section of this book if plain water is unappetizing. As part of your daily water intake, each morning, start your day off with a cup of hot water with freshly squeezed lemon juice from half of a lemon.

Steer clear of all corn, beans, soy, wheat and dairy products. *Essentially, any foods on the approved list with a (*) are off limits during this time.* Frankly, you should be limiting these foods anyway as regular consumption will not contribute to optimal health. But for the sake of not feeling deprived, you may eliminate these for the short one to three weeks to cleanse your body.

Eliminate your cheat foods (all alcohol, chocolate, sweets, etc.) during this time. Also, eat only super pure fats (i.e., avocado, coconut oil, olive oil, etc.) and avoid nuts, seeds, and nut butter for now. Some folks find that overeating nut butter or nuts will prevent weight loss and cause water retention.

Remember, once you have given yourself a break, you can always go back to healthy servings of them. But for now, stick to your guns and member "why" you wish to give your body a break to cleanse and rejuvenate.

Make sure that you are not ingesting any pesticides that are creating a burden on your liver. The more toxicity you have, the less effective your fat loss will be. Take advantage of additional liver support by drinking a detoxifying tea or taking supplementation suggested to you by your healthcare provider (see **Daily Detoxification** for extra help to support your week(s) of cleansing).

If you have a mini trampoline, make sure to jump 10-20 minutes per day to move your lymphatic system. Otherwise, find time to do yoga with deep breathing (ujjayi pranayama) and plenty of inversions and twisting poses for detoxifying your organs. And don't forget to find ways to de-stress. Make sure you follow the tips listed in **Reassess Your Stress Levels**, located in the chapter, **Breaking the Plateau.** De-stressing doesn't have to be complicated; but, it does need to be nurturing and assist you in letting go of tension. It should be something that you look forward to doing each day during this cleansing process.

In the next couple of chapters, you will determine which side of the camp you are currently on: higher carbohydrate intake or lower carbohydrate intake. If you are eating around 150 grams or less of carbs per day, you may be in the lower carb camp. Conversely, if you are eating over 200 grams of carbohydrates per day, you are in the higher carb intake camp. If you don't know where you are, I suggest you track your eating habits on the My Fitness Pal or Cronometer phone app for three days. Tracking your food for three days will give you a good idea where you need to start. If you are a high carb person, currently, start with the chapter, **From High Carb to Low Carb**. If you are low carb, skip to **Low Carbohydrate Lifestyle, Already?**

Chapter 6

From High Carb to Low Carb
Assisting You with the Transition

Once you have cleared your pantry, cupboards, and refrigerator of all the foods with ingredients listed in the previous paragraphs, then you are ready to start your new lifestyle and dietary journey. It is important to note that while some people like to jump in right away and go "all in" to a low carbohydrate and higher fat lifestyle, there are some things you must consider.

First, if you have been eating foods with sugar and like your oatmeal or cereal for breakfast, your sandwiches for lunch, your rice and pasta dishes for dinner, etc. then you can be assured that you are burning primarily glucose as your fuel source. While the body is an incredible machine and can switch from glucose to fat as fuel, this adjustment takes some time. Not only does it take time; but, the body can go through "withdrawal" and folks who make this transition may experience what some like to call "the carb flu." Symptoms can include agitated mood, low energy, headaches, body aches, hunger pangs, etc. Sounds fun, right? Yeah, not so much. I know because I have experienced this and at first it seemed to be the flu; but, after putting two and two together it was apparent I was going through the "fat adaptation" as some call it.

Now before you freak out and say, "I'm not doing this. Why would I want to go through that?" please understand — that first, it is temporary and you feel *fantastic* on the other side. Also, it is important to note that you don't have to go through this process if you take it slow and follow some of these helpful tips and tricks that I have since learned from experiencing the "carb flu." If you have had a carbohydrate-driven diet (even if you are paleo or primal in your eating habits), then you will need to prepare yourself by choosing one of two options:

1) Ease into the diet guidelines I have outlined for you. You will ease into them by allowing yourself some healthy substitutions for your current carb-laden foods. Skim through **The Plan: Approved Foods** to get an idea of the foods list you will be using for your transition. Allow yourself to have two full servings of fruit per day, two full servings of an approved carbohydrate and two cheats per day. Technically, you may choose to have six servings of carbohydrate-packed food to help you transition from your sugar cravings to a more nutritional fat-adapted, lower carbohydrate diet, if you desire.

2) OR, you can choose to jump into the diet and utilize nutritional support to alleviate some of the common symptoms, avoid the "flu" and get started on a low-

er carbohydrate diet right away. I only suggest this method if you have been eating a Paleo-style diet and looking to decrease your carbohydrate content. Skim through **The Plan: Approved Foods** to get an idea of the foods list you will be using for your transition. Whether you choose the first option or the second option, you must listen to your body and any signs that you need to make adjustments in your macronutrients. You can review these indications in **The Plan: Calculate Your Caloric Needs.**

I'm not going to determine what is best for you. Only you will know what you are willing and able to do. However, if you choose option #1, then here is a template to follow. Review my recipes to find some that have the carbohydrates that interest you and plan to have the ingredients handy as you prepare for your transition to a lower carb lifestyle.

Option #1
Week One

Start with two servings of fruit (I suggest that for this purpose a serving size is a large granny smith apple and one cup of berries). Eat two servings of complex carbohydrates (I recommend 1/2 cup of sweet potato, quinoa, plantain or almond flour). Indulge in two approved treats per day (1 oz of 85% dark chocolate or 5 oz of dry red wine). So, for example, you may choose to have 2 cups of berries, 1 cup of roasted sweet potato, one ounce of chocolate and

5 oz of wine, each day. Also, start increasing your fat content incrementally. The idea here is to gradually start adding in more fat to your diet to help keep you satiated without overloading your stomach, gall bladder, pancreas, etc. You need to prepare these organs with the necessary bile and enzymes to break down the fat. If you experience issues with your digestion, drop the servings of fat and consider taking bile salts or pancreatic enzymes. Add one TBL of coconut oil to your food each day. Eat at least one-half of a whole avocado per day and feel free to put grass-fed butter on your vegetables. Don't count calories right now. You may gain a little weight, and this is ok. It will come back off, over time as you adjust to your new eating plan. Do this for one week. Aim for four servings of dark green leafy veggies per day. You can make a green shake if this is easier for you (see recipes). Drink two liters of water per day or eight cups.

Week Two

This week you will have two servings of fruit, again. You will have one serving of complex carbohydrate (1/2 cup) and 1 treat every day of the week. This week increase your fat intake by adding in another tablespoon of coconut oil (2 total) each day. Eat one avocado per day. Feel free to smother your roasted veggies in grass-fed butter. The idea here is to incrementally start adding more fat to your diet to help keep you satiated without overloading your stomach, gallbladder, pancreas, etc. You need to prepare these organs with the necessary bile and enzymes to break down the fat. Aim for

6 (six) servings of dark green leafy veggies per day. Drink three liters of water per day or 12 cups.

Week Three

Continue to eat your two servings of fruit. You will have one serving of complex carbohydrate, and you will have one treat, 3x this week. Choose the days that you want to schedule your treats. This week increase your fat intake by adding in another one tablespoon of coconut oil (3 total) per day. Eat one whole avocado per day and smother your roasted veggies in grass-fed butter. You can have as much fat as you want right now; but, be mindful of your digestion and how your body responds to the added fats. If you experience issues with your digestion, drop the servings of fat and consider taking bile salts or pancreatic enzymes. Aim for eight servings of dark green leafy veggies per day. Drink four liters of water per day or 16 cups.

Week Four

Week four is your final week of transition. Continue with your two servings of fruit. Decrease your complex carbohydrates to 1/4 cup or 1/2 serving of complex carbohydrate each day. Then you will have one day that you will have a treat. This week increase your fat intake by adding in another 1 TBL of coconut (4 total) oil per day. Eat one whole avocado per day and smother your roasted veggies in grass-fed butter. You can have as much fat as you want right now; but, be mindful of your digestion and how your body responds to the added fats. If you experience issues with your digestion, drop the servings of fat and consider taking bile salts or pancreatic enzymes. Continue to let yourself have AS MUCH fat as you want. Aim for ten dark green leafy veggies per day. Continue to drink four liters or 16 cups of water (or more) per day.

Once you complete this week, you will be ready to transition into your new diet plan. You may choose to start the nutrition program with two servings of fruit and no complex carbohydrates. However, even after completing this Option #1 process, I suggest you read all of **The Plan Calculate your Caloric Needs** to review how to make adjustments in your fat and carbohydrate servings based on your cravings, energy, hunger, sleep patterns, mood and exercise performance. If you determine that you feel great going very low carbohydrate and none of these indicators have signaled an imbalance in your system, then you can try very low carbohydrate. Use any and all of Option #2 guidelines. These will be necessary for you, even if you had success with option #1.

Option #2

If you chose this as your option to jump right into a lower carbohydrate diet, then I congratulate you on your enthusiasm and fervor. Use the guidelines outlined in this section, in conjunction with the diet guidelines provided in **The Plan Approved Foods** and **The Plan: Calculate Your Caloric Needs.** Know that while you may have some difficulty at first, the symptoms usually pass after a few days—and, in most healthy individuals, the transition is *usual-*

ly fully complete in a matter of a couple of weeks and one is in full-fat burning mode once fully "adapted" to the lower carbohydrate intake. Please be patient. Depending on your overall health, the process could take longer and upwards of a couple of months. For some folks, adaptation can take up to a year, if they are not metabolically sound or their hormones are imbalanced. Remember, from a previous chapter, that losing weight is not nearly as much about caloric intake as it is hormone balance! The truth that weight loss is not always about calories in and calories out is why I suggest you see a holistic practitioner to get tested and treated for any imbalances before embarking on dietary changes.

To help you mitigate some of the symptoms that people often experience and make it as easy as possible, I'll provide you will some helpful tools for starting your lower carbohydrate journey. The reason for a lot of the symptoms in transitioning from carbohydrate and sugar burning to fat burning has a lot to do with the body's adjustment to electrolyte balance. What? Yeah, believe it or not, when you eat carbohydrates and sugar, your body retains water and easily keeps electrolytes (think sodium, potassium, magnesium, etc.). Given this fact, there is an immediate dropping of water weight when you start a lower carbohydrate diet. With this flushing of excess water, your body expels your much-needed electrolytes.

This flushing of electrolytes can be easily mitigated by adding 1-2 Tsp of salt per day to your food or water and eating a ton of green veggies. Aim for 10 cups of dark leafy greens, green powders, and cruciferous vegetables, per day! Adding a potassium citrate supplement to your regimen and eating lots of avocados in the beginning stages, is very helpful. Get plenty of B vitamins as this is crucial. If you are not sensitive to egg yolks, these are high in B vitamins. A multi B vitamin to assist your adrenals in adjusting to the new electrolyte balance will be extremely helpful, also. Make sure that it is high in pantothenic acid (B5). Take one in the am with food and one in the afternoon with food. I like Integrative Therapeutics multi B supplement. Increase your magnesium supplementation and eat raw cacao and the approved servings of nuts and nut butter. Don't forget that it is imperative that you rehydrate your body. Shoot for drinking your total body weight in ounces of water. Check out my water recipes for creative ways to make water taste better!

Adding vitamin and mineral-rich foods and electrolyte supplementation as you transition into your new dietary habits will be beneficial in alleviating any common symptoms people experience, otherwise. It is important to note that you must have healthy kidney function and you must be cleared by your physician before you make significant changes to your diet or supplement regimen.

You've Done Option #1 or #2, Now What?

Once you have made it through one or both of the above options, you are ready to move on to the prescribed diet plan. You should be starting the program feeling rather comfortable with two servings of fruit and between zero and two servings of complex carbohydrates, depending on how your body feels. If you haven't done so already, jump ahead to **The Plan: The Approved Foods**, to become familiar with what foods you should have stocked in your pantry and refrigerator. Then, in The Plan: Calculate Your Caloric Needs, you will learn how to make the necessary adjustments to your diet to make this plan your own; your personalized program for fat loss. Are you as excited as I am? Now, it is time to dive deep and explore how you are going to adopt a new lifestyle and new eating habits.

Chapter 7

Low Carbohydrate Lifestyle, Already?

Transition into Your Maintenance Program or Continue Fat Loss

Some folks who read this book may already be on a low carb diet, a moderate carb diet or have a history of carbohydrate restriction. Some folks may have tried a medically supervised diet program for weight loss utilizing hCG (human chorionic gonadotropin) and are now looking for a method to maintain their new weight or continue to lose weight if that is their goal. This book is the perfect assistance for maintaining or continuing weight loss after hCG programs. However, before you consider hCG, make sure you find a practitioner who is interested in reviewing laboratory work, requires a full patient intake and who assesses your overall metabolic status before prescribing it.

If you have started to decrease your carbohydrates in any fashion, then this book will be very beneficial for you in maintaining your weight loss as well as learning how to incorporate variety into your diet appropriately without sabotaging your results. As a measure of ensuring success, it is imperative that you carefully integrate new foods into your diet with precision and strategy. When a plan for food implementation is not present, one is more inclined to put guess work into their dietary habits —and thus, is set up for self-sabotage and a frustrating journey toward weight gain.

The transition from low carbohydrate to a more fat-friendly (fat for fuel, rather than glucose) lifestyle is crucial, and those who are interested in maintaining their weight loss should consider remaining on a low carbohydrate, moderate protein, and higher fat diet to sustain the benefits. If you choose a more ketogenic approach (very low carbohydrate and higher fat intake), I suggest that you research the ketogenic diet further. An excellent web page to visit: http://biohackingwellness.com/mighty-mitochondria/ to get great tips on how this lifestyle can benefit you.

Also, drinking 100 oz minimum of water; adding in physical activity at this point and maintaining a caloric range for stabilization of their new weight or continual weight loss is crucial to one's success.

In the beginning, it is necessary to introduce more fats and protein sources with a decrease in carbohydrate intake and—only if one chooses to, very slowly add some of the options for complex carbohydrates (only green approved food options), to tolerance. However, this process must be calculated and purposeful for success to occur. The mistake that many people make at this point is adding in too much, too soon. Doing so can often add on pounds that folks have worked so hard to shed.

Also, *if you have been at a caloric deficit, you will need to slowly add in calories every week until you reach the suggested calculation that is best for you as described in* **The Plan: Calculate Your Caloric Needs**. If you don't know if you are at a caloric deficit, compare what you are eating now (by tracking your food in My Fitness Pal) and comparing this number to the maintenance number in **The Plan: Calculate Your Caloric Needs**. So, for example, if you have been eating 1400 calorie for a while and you calculate in **The Plan Calculate Your Caloric Needs** that maintenance is 2,300 calories, then you are at a 900 caloric deficit. If you ascertain that weight loss will require approximately 1,700 calories per day, then you ought to slowly add calories each week until you hit this number. I suggest adding 50-100 calories per day for one week. Add 100 calories each week until you reach your target number of calories. This way, you give the body a chance to adapt to the change and prevent any "freaking out" or rebound weight gain.

As you track your reactions to food, you can utilize the **Food and Reaction Tracker** from journeytowardjoy.com in the menu tab labeled "Resources." I suggest that if you are transitioning from a strict low carbohydrate diet, that you follow these guidelines to safely introduce fun food and safe carbohydrates:

Week One:

Add in *one* serving of nuts, seeds or nut butter (i.e., 24 almonds) and continue to get the remaining fat servings from coconut oil, avocado oil, avocado, MCT oil, etc. The key is to pay attention to all of your body's hormonal responses and reactions to food. Indicators that you need to back away from a recently introduced food group can include: weight gain the next day (a result of inflammation and water retention), poor digestion (bloating, gas), decreased energy, increased cravings, disturbances in sleep, changes in mood and affect, etc. You can use the Food and Reactions Tracker at journeytowardjoy.com if you need a print out to assist you. Any of these signs can indicate that you are *not* ready for the reintroduction of nuts or seeds—and therefore, you should abstain. Once you test nuts with your constitution and determine if your body is ready for consumption, then I suggest that for *one* of the days this first week, you also add in 5 oz of **very dry** red wine (no more). You can find my red wine suggestions in the **Recipes** section of this book.

Again, it is important to check your weight the next day in conjunction with diligently monitoring all of the indicators mentioned above. Any fluctuation in weight (upwards) or changes in digestion energy, cravings, sleep, mood and workout performance is an indicator that you are too sensitive to alcohol and you should abstain, for now. If your weight does not increase after your 5 oz intake of wine, then may allow yourself to indulge up to 2 (two) 5 oz glasses at a time, in one day. However, know that with every glass of wine, you run the risk of halting the breakdown of fat in your body up to 24-48 hours. Therefore, it is my recommendation that if you are going to indulge, do so only ONCE per week, to maintain continual fat burning. An additional tip worth mentioning: if you drink wine, do so without fat or carbohydrates at your meal or drink it alone away from any food. In the presence of carbohydrates or fat, your body will always prefer detoxification to fat burning. Your meal most likely will end up stored, rather than burned, if you combine alcohol with fat and carbohydrates. Boo!! I know, you will thank me later. An early "You're welcome!" to you!

Also, you may try to have 1 oz of dark (85% or higher) chocolate. Do this on a day you do not have wine or nuts, so that you can monitor any fluctuations in weight or in the indicators that you are tracking each day. If you can tolerate chocolate, then this is a healthful "cheat" for you to have on a regular basis.

If you choose not to have wine or chocolate, then continue to have two servings of fruit per day. This week, you are not taking in any additional complex carbohydrates except for fruit, wine or chocolate. See **The Plan: Approved Foods** for ideas of allowed foods to have.

Once you determine if your body is adaptable to one serving of nuts, wine, and chocolate, then you are ready to try complex carbohydrates in Week Two. However, if you are satisfied with nuts, wine and chocolate and you do not wish to add complex carbohydrates, then feel free to move onto the next chapter. If your body negatively reacted to any of these three items, then it is important to note that you will need to refrain for quite a while. For certain body constitutions, this may mean six months or a year, it depends. If you have a food sensitivity, then you may need to refrain from these foods inevitably based on your constitution.

Please note that the key here is to pay attention to your reactions to food and abstain from those things that are preventing you from obtaining your ideal health and physique. It is my preference that folks remain eating in this style as their lifestyle diet of choice or at least give it a try for a minimum of 2 (two) months to see how their body responds. Ultimately, the diet is around 30-70% fat, 5-30% carbohydrate and 20-40% protein, depending upon your body's needs. This method of eating has provided significant strides in my overall well-being and blood markers from my laboratory results —but, not just me. In fact, it has benefitted many with whom I consult.

Given these results, it is imperative to note; some individuals will benefit from having complex carbohydrates in their diet. The variance in individual response to carb intake is why the percentages for each macronutrient are so varied. Take responsibility and do the proper investigation to determine where your body finds hormonal balance. In the case of adrenal stress, hormonal imbalance, some "weight loss plateaus," or for very active people, adding in the allowed serving of carbohydrates is necessary to maintain healthy energy, appetite, sleep, and athletic performance. While these exceptions tend to be rarer than the general public would like to believe, it happens, and these individuals will improve their sense of well-being and address imbalance with the right combination of fruits and complex carbohydrates. How do you determine how much you need? You have to start slowly and add in a little at a time as suggested in the following paragraphs.

If you have been on a low carbohydrate diet for a long time and your weight loss has stalled, your workouts are suffering, or your sleep patterns are disrupted, then going very low carb may not be the best choice for you. Start with the approved two servings of fruit and then play around with slowly integrating complex carbohydrates. You can start with week 2 and see how you feel. If you feel noticeably better, you can stay at this point for a while. Pay attention to all of the indicators of hormonal imbalance (weight gain, decreased energy, cravings, sleep disturbance, changes in mood/affect and decreased workout performance). If you move up to week 3 and don't feel as well, then move back to week 2. You can use this method for any level outlined below. Frankly, you should stay where you feel the best and back down if you don't. It is that simple.

You may not be in ketosis if you incorporate fruit and complex carbohydrates; but, that is alright. You can try ketosis in the future, if you wish, by eliminating fruits and complex carbohydrate foods and following the plan outlined in the chapter, **From High Carb to Low Carb**. However, I do not recommend that you go too low in carbohydrates if you have any signs of hormonal imbalance. Trust me, I know. Where you start or where you feel the best often depends on your state of hormonal balance, your activity levels, and your stress levels. If weight loss is your goal, remember that hormones will determine your rate of weight loss more than your caloric intake! Therefore, you must follow your body's lead when it comes to indicators that it is not ready for drastic changes.

For some, going into full ketosis will be too much of a stressor on the body, and the adrenals will raise cortisol levels, resulting in higher blood glucose. Elevated blood glucose will negate the effects one may be trying to achieve. So, do the body a favor and pay attention to the signs that the body is stressed, imbalanced, etc. Even better, get your levels tested (Adrenal Stress Index, a DUTCH Hormone and adrenal panel, etc.). If you suspect that you need a bit more carbohydrates in your diet based on your symptom picture or your laboratory tests, then, you may want to follow the weekly plan, outlined below, to help you nourish your body without overdoing it or sabotaging your health-related goals.

Week Two:

Add in a half of one serving of complex carbohydrate (i.e., 1/4 cup of squash, almond flour or the green carbohydrate foods, etc.) for one day. Pay attention to all of your body's hormonal responses and reactions to food. Indicators that you need to back away from a recently introduced food group can include: weight gain the next day (a result of inflammation and water retention), poor digestion (bloating, gas), decreased energy, increased cravings, disturbances in sleep, changes in mood and affect, etc. You can use the Food and Reactions Tracker at journeytowardjoy.com if you need a print out to assist you. Any of these signs can indicate that you are *not* ready for the reintroduction of complex carbohydrates, yet. Stick to the plan outlined in Week One and move on to **The Plan: Calculate Your Caloric Needs.** Otherwise, if you did not experience any unfavorable changes and you can tolerate a half serving of complex carbohydrate, then move on to week three.

Week Three:

Have one whole serving of green complex carbohydrate per day, noting any adverse changes in your hormonal indicators as discussed in previous weeks. If you experience any negative symptoms, then go back to week two, having only half a serving. Keep your servings of nuts and seeds to one per day, your wine intake to one day per week and try a dose of dark chocolate (1 oz) on the days you do not have wine and in place of the one serving of complex carbohydrate or fruit. You may move on to **The Plan: Calculate Your Caloric Needs.** If you are free of any negative signs that hormones are out of balance, then move on to week four.

Week Four:

Have one and one-half servings of green complex carbohydrates noting any adverse changes in your hormonal indicators as discussed in previous weeks. If you experience any negative signs, then go back to week three, having only one serving. Keep your servings of nuts and seeds to one per day, your wine intake to one day per week and try a dose of dark chocolate (1 oz) on the days you do not have wine and in place of the one serving of complex carbohydrate or fruit. You may move onto **The Plan: Calculate Your Caloric Needs.** If you are free of any negative signs that hormones are out of balance, then move onto week five.

Week Five:

Have two servings of green complex carbohydrates noting any adverse changes in your hormonal indicators as discussed in previous weeks. If you experience any negative signs, then go back to week four, having only one and a half serving. Keep your servings of nuts and seeds to one per day, your wine intake to one day per week and try a dose of dark chocolate (1 oz) on the days you do not have wine and in place of the one serving of complex carbohydrate or fruit. You may move on to **The Plan: Calculate Your Caloric Needs.** If you are free of any negative signs that hormones are out of balance, then you may keep your two servings of complex carbohydrates and move on to week five.

What Now???

Whether you moved up to week five or you stayed at week one, you now know how your body reacts to the addition of some of the allowed carbohydrates and "cheats." Because you now have this information, you are ready to follow the nutrition guide and suggested servings of **The Plan**.

PART 2
THE PLAN

Chapter 8

The Plan: Approved Foods

Easy Guide For Making Better Choices

This chapter offers a comprehensive list of approved foods except for a few that should be limited **(*).** Simplifying the process further for you requires making you aware of a few key things.

> TIP:
>
> ***It is important to note that the printed version of this book is in black and white; therefore, for any color-coding (i.e. approved foods list) see the Kindle version (by downloading the Kindle application on your device) or visit my webpage: journeyto-wardjoy.com and click on the Resources tab.*

First, I have provided a list of **LOW GLYCEMIC (1-55)** foods (in green) that will allow you to choose items that won't spike your blood sugar levels. By preventing a spike in blood sugar, you prevent a spiking of insulin —and thus, keep insulin under control. Choosing foods that are low glycemic means that you are less likely to develop insulin resistance, inflammation, and the mental and energetic crashes that come from glucose dysregulation. But, to take it step further, foods at the top of each list, (in green), are not only low on the glycemic index; but they are low on the **INSULIN INDEX.**

Why is this important? While the Glycemic Index (GI) is a measurement of the sugar response in the blood (how fast carbohydrates turn into or affect blood sugars), the Insulin Index (II) measures how foods, *including non-carbohydrate* foods, will trigger insulin. Because insulin lowers blood sugar by shuttling it into the cells, as long as insulin is spiked (or present), it is nearly impossible to be in fat burning mode, whatsoever. So, if your goal is to burn fat, then paying attention to the Insulin Index, will be essential to your success. Foods that have a cautionary level or **MEDIUM GLYCEMIC (56-69)** or have a medium effect on your insulin levels are highlighted in yellow or remain **black**. And, the foods that you should limit as much as possible because they are **HIGH GLYCEMIC (70-100)** or that spike your insulin levels—and are higher on the II—should be limited and are highlighted in red. It doesn't mean that you can't ever have these foods; however, you should aim for no more than once per week, unless you are a vegetarian, vegan, etc.

In addition to monitoring your blood sugar, the goal in creating this guided food list is to assist you in choosing foods that optimize your overall nutrition and metabolic function. Choosing foods that are higher alkaline forming (in green, again) will help you create a minimized acidic environment in your body—which means that bacteria, viruses, cancer cells, etc. are less likely to thrive and grow. Foods that are highlighted in yellow or remain **black** are less alkaline forming or more neutral. These foods are safe, but for optimum health shoot for getting the majority of your foods that are green. So, ultimately, the more green foods you have, the better your overall health and vitality. Keep in mind, that for weight loss, the insulin index will trump all other factors, so stick to mostly green and occasional black foods, and you'll be safe.

We all know that decreasing the toxic load with eating more clean, fresh, organic food is necessary. However, if you are on a budget or you need to know what foods you should buy organic, I have labeled these for you. Look for **(H)** for the foods that are high pesticide risk. Whenever possible, buy the organic form. Low pesticide risk is labeled with **(L)** and indicates that it is relatively safe to buy the regular forms of these foods over the more expensive organic varieties.

TIP:

If you have limited access to organic fruits and vegetables or you have a limited budget, you can do a "wash" in your kitchen sink with one of four methods. 1) Put the food in your kitchen sink half filled with water and one tsp of castile soap. Then scrub your produce with a veggie brush. 2) Add 1 TBL of 35% hydrogen peroxide to a kitchen sink half full of water and let soak for 5-15 minutes (longer for thicker skins) Rinse very well. 3) Add one tsp of Clorox bleach to a gallon of water and soak your

produce for 5-15 minutes (again, use the longer
time for thicker skins). Do not use any other brand
as many have harmful chemicals added. Rinse very
well. 4) Use one part vinegar to three parts water.
All of these options will help to kill bacteria and
keep your veggies and fruit fresher, longer.

Lastly, when you see a food item with a (*) next to it, this is something you should limit in your diet. These are items that — if eaten too often, may not contribute to your overall health and wellness. Because this book is *not* about deprivation, if you love these foods, then choose to enjoy the highest quality form you can find, on occasion. Just don't go crazy and have these foods every day. If you are a vegetarian or vegan, then allow yourself to partake in eating the listed foods, including those labeled (*) to suit your needs.

Vegetables:

All non-starchy vegetables are fair game. There are no limits on serving size or amount; however, always aim for a minimum of your daily servings required (see **The Plan: Calculate Your Caloric Needs**). A serving size is typically 1 cup unless otherwise specified. Whenever possible, buy only organic when selecting leafy greens or vegetables with soft skins. With tougher skins, you can be less strict as previously mentioned. As noted in previous chapters of this book, you should aim for ten servings per day (especially of the dark green leafy varieties).

Horseradish

Asparagus (L) (10 spears)

Celery (H)

All green leafy vegetables raw (H) (1/2 cup cooked)

Beet greens

Spinach (H)

Bell pepper (H)

Broccoli

Cabbage (L)

Kale (H)

Daikon

Mushrooms (L)

Cucumber (H)

Cauliflower (L)

Sprouts

Brussel sprouts (5 medium)

Tomatoes (H) (2 medium)

Artichokes (1/2 large)

Onions (L)

*Peas (L)

*Corn on the cob (L)

*Carrots (10 medium baby carrots or 1 cup sliced regular)

*Beets (2 medium)

TIP:

(*) These foods are higher in carbohydrates, so limit these to no more than one serving per day to keep sugars at bay.

Fruits:

A serving size is 3/4 cup (sliced if a non-berry fruit) or 1 whole unless specified. If you are working toward a very low carbohydrate lifestyle, then you may choose to eliminate fruit for now. If you decide to remove fruit, you can slowly add fruit (one to two servings per day) back into your diet once you reach your preferred maintenance weight. When you start eating fruit again, it is best to stick to the green fruits. Fruit other than the green items below will spike insulin a bit more.

Lemons (L)

Limes (L)

Raspberries (H)

Blackberries (H)

Strawberries (H)

Pear (H)

Mango (L)

Grapes (H)

Kiwi (L) (2 small)

Apples (H)

Berries

Dates (2 small)

Grapefruit (L) (1/2 of a large)

Peaches (H)

Blueberries (H)

Boysenberries (H)

Apricot (H) (4 small)

Cantaloupe (L)

Dried Figs

Pineapple (L)

Cherries

Fresh figs

Bananas (L) (1/2 of medium size)

Oranges (L) (medium size)

Papaya (L)

Raisins (H)

Watermelon

TIP:

Fruits with tough skin have lower pesticide risk.
However, when it comes to fruits with a soft skin,
you should opt for organic, as much as possible.

Meat and Protein:

A serving size is 3/4 cup or 4-6 oz unless otherwise specified.
When purchasing seafood, buy wild caught fish. When picking out
meat, poultry and eggs, buy certified organic, free-range (pasture-
raised is great) and humanely certified items, as much as possible.

Minimize all dairy products in your daily intake. If you choose to eat dairy, make sure that is organic and of the highest quality that you can afford. Look for meat and dairy products that are hormone, pesticide, antibiotic and cruelty-free. After all, any toxicity in the products that you consume becomes your toxicity issue. You don't want any added toxicity if you are trying to adopt a clean and healthful lifestyle. Quality matters! So, if you are a meat eater, please vote with your wallet and support the humane treatment of animals and the growth of organic farms!

Sardines (7 medium)
Herring
Anchovies
Mackerel
Mahimahi
Halibut
White sea bass
Trout
Bacon
Duck
Tuna, fresh
Eggs (2 large, whole)
Grass-fed beef (grass-finished if you can find it)
Chicken
Ground chicken or turkey
Lamb
Pork
Salmon

Tuna canned (limited)

Protein powder (15-21 grams of protein, preferably pea or hemp)

*Tempeh (organic, non-GMO)

*Tofu (organic, non-GMO)

*Greek yogurt (full fat, plain)

*Cottage cheese (full-fat)

Egg whites (8 large)

Shellfish (oysters, crab, scallops, lobster, clam mussels)

*Whey protein

*Greek yogurt plain 1 or 2%

*Cottage cheese 2%

> **TIP:**
>
> *Unless you are vegetarian or vegan, limit these foods to no more than one serving (in total) per day. Ideally, you will only partake on a rare occasion. Vegans will want to amplify their protein intake with supplemental protein powders and plant-based sources.*

Starchy Complex Carbohydrates:

A serving size is 1/2 cup unless otherwise specified. NOTE: If you are just starting out on this journey and you have been relying on carbs and sugars for fuel, then you will want to start off your diet first by following the suggestions outlined in Option #1 of **From High Carb to Low Carb**. This plan will ease you into the lower carbohydrate lifestyle. When you are ready, limit yourself to one to two servings of the green foods. For the black choices, aim to have these on occasion.

Almond flour (1/4 cup—it is recommended that you limit almond flour to one serving per day)

Unsweetened almond, hemp, coconut milk (from a carton, not canned, 2 cups)

Zucchini squash

Summer squash (H)

Pumpkin squash

Quinoa cooked

Sweet potato (L)

Yams (L)

Plantain (sliced)

Squash (butternut, spaghetti, etc.)

Coconut water (2 cups)

Tapioca flour(1/4 cup)

Coconut flour (1/4 cup)

*Edamame

*Oatmeal steel cut

*Cow's milk, whole (1 cup)

*Beans cooked

*Sweet corn on the cob (1 ear)

*Lentils

*Bread (whole grain sprouted one slice)

*Wild rice

    TIP:

Limit these items. The foods labeled with ""
should not be eaten every day as they can cause insulin and glucose dysregulation. The exceptions are
beans and lentils. When eating these legumes, make
sure they are soaked properly for at least 24 hours
before cooking and serving. One to two servings of
these per day will not spike your blood glucose levels too much and are a great protein source for veg-
ans. Otherwise, if you choose to have the (*) items,
do so infrequently. For optimum health, I suggest
you attempt to avoid dairy and grains, altogether.*

Healthful Fats:

A serving size is 1/4 cup.

Avocado (L) mashed or 1/4 of a LARGE
Coconut (unsweetened, shaved)
Canned coconut milk (full-fat)
Coconut cream
Almond flour (limit almond flour to one serving in a day)
Olives (20-count)
*Full-fat cream
*Shredded cheese (full-fat)
*Goat cheese
*Buttermilk
*Hummus

Nuts and Seeds:

Raw nuts (limit to 1 oz *per* day): *A serving size for each type of nut is specified:*

24 raw almonds, 20 pecan halves, 28 whole peanuts, 14 walnut halves, 12 macadamia nuts, eight brazil nuts, 16 cashews, 45 whole pistachios, 167 pine nuts

Raw seeds (2 TBL of the following):

pumpkin, chia, flax, sesame, sunflower, hemp, etc.

Oils and Butters:

Olive oil (1 TBL)
Coconut oil (1 TBL)
Avocado oil (1TBL)
Kerrygold butter (1 TBL)
Nut butter (limit to 1 serving per day): almond, peanut, coconut, cashew (2 TBL)
Seed butter (limit to 1 serving per day): Sesame/tahini, pumpkin, etc. (2 TBL)
Homemade salad dressing or mayonnaise (2 TBL)

Most store-bought salad dressings are full of fillers and ingredients that will not assist you in your journey toward better health. Start learning to make homemade dressings in large batches and always have some handy. Do not purchase nut butter that has more ingredients listed than nuts and salt. Any hydrogenated fats, fillers, sugars, etc. are a hindrance to your overall health. While nuts and nut butter are delicious, try not to go overboard with these and measure out your servings. Too much, for some people, can stall weight loss.

Healthful "Cheats":

These are fun food items are optional. You can have one or two chocolate "cheats" per day, but I highly suggest that you avoid having red wine every night if you are serious about fat burning. While it has many health benefits and is one of my favorite splurges, you run the risk of kicking your body out of fat burning mode — and while it is temporary, if drunk every day, most folks will not make significant progress in their weight loss. Also, for each serving of an allowed cheat (up to two) in one day, you must eliminate a serving of fruit or complex carbohydrate that day.

1 oz of 85% or higher dark chocolate (bonus points if you choose stevia-sweetened chocolate bars found at most natural health food stores).

*5-6 oz of red wine (1-2 servings on one night of the week)

TIP:

*If you want to lose weight, I suggest no more than two servings of wine or alcohol per week and that you have them on THE SAME NIGHT. Alcohol can stall fat burning for 24-48 hours, so if you are serious about weight loss, cut down on your booze. If you are sensitive to sulfites, try wines from Heartswork Winery, such as Well Red or try Roule Rouge (both are available at Trader Joes) as neither wine has added sulfites and are certified low in sulfites. Also, a Paleo friendly wine acclaimed for being free of headaches and hangovers is Dry Farms Wines. You can purchase both reds and whites (and bubbly) from their web page **dry-farmwines.com.** Another option is Fit Vine Wines. Their wine is biodynamically processed, has no residual sugar and is "headache-free." Bonus: only 95 calories for a 5 oz glass. You can purchase a bottle to try at **fitvinewines.com**. As mentioned in a previous chapter, it is best to drink wine without fat or carbohydrates at your meal or to drink it alone away from any food. In the presence of carbohy-*

drates or fat, your body will always prefer detoxifi-
cation to fat burning. Your meal most likely will end
up stored, rather than burned, if you combine alco-
hol with fat and carbohydrates.

Free Foods:

Green tea

Apple cider vinegar

Ginger root

Sweeteners such as stevia (I recommend flavored sweet leaf stevia drops), monk fruit (Luo Han Guo) and Xylitol. Some people are sensitive to the digestive effects of sugar alcohols, so be careful with any sugar ending in "ol" such as maltitol, erythritol, etc. While these are allowed, some folks experience digestion distress (you know, like gas and bloating...the socially fun ones).

All spices

All herbs fresh and dried

Tea and coffee (move toward decaffeinated, organic, fair trade, etc.)

Vinegars

Mustard

Hot sauce

Pure extracts (vanilla, almond, etc.)

Chapter 9

The Plan: Calculate Your Caloric Needs

How to Customize Your Individual Plan

Now it is time for us to move on to the details for determining how you will optimize your nutrition and reach your overall wellness goals. The steps I have provided for you below will get you well on your way to start your new journey.

Use your current weight to determine your caloric needs. Your caloric range will be adjusted as your weight changes with eating and exercise so refer to this page often as your weight fluctuates up or down.

STEP 1:

Multiply your current weight times your current activity level. If you are sedentary or have a desk job, multiply your weight X 11. If you do light housework and are on your feet for part of the day, multiply your weight X 12. If you have a manual labor job or are on your feet all day, multiply your weight X 13. If you are sedentary (which will hopefully change soon), then *stick with the number you have calculated for step 1 as your caloric range*. If you are an active individual, move on to step 2.

STEP 2:

Add 450 to the number calculated in step 1. If you are attempting to maintain your weight, then this is your final number. If you wish to lose weight, then move to step number 3. HOWEVER...IF YOU HAVE BEEN A CHRONIC DIETER AND HAVE BEEN AT A CALORIC DEFICIT FOR A WHILE, AND HAVE EXPERIENCED A LENGTHY PLATEAU, PLEASE DO YOUR BODY A FAVOR AND STOP HERE! Your body will most likely not respond to a caloric deficit at this point if you have been chronically dieting. Your metabolism may be slow as a result; and therefore, by continuing to cut calories, you may not experience further weight loss, right now. Thus, you will need to eat at maintenance for a while and heal your metabolism. Trust me. The signals that you are free to cut back on your calories (within reason) will be: your sleep, energy, cravings, digestion, mood and workout performance are on point (discussed later in this chapter). Then *and only then*, may you move on to step three. For some, *this may take a few months*. But, you have to understand that weight loss *cannot* be a quick fix. You must heal the body for your ultimate health to occur. It will seem like too many calories for some folks; but, many folks start to lose weight once they feed their body the energy that it needs. As a method of getting to this number, I suggest adding 50-100 calories to your current caloric intake, for one week. So, for example, if you currently eat 1,400 calories, then for one week, eat 1,500. Each subsequent week add 50-100 calories until you reach your target maintenance number. This way, you give the body a chance to adapt to the change and prevent any "freaking out" or rebound weight gain. When you reach maintenance, stay at this number for one to two months to heal your metabolism. Then, you may move on to step 3.

STEP 3:

Subtract 200-300 from the number calculated in step 2. If your final number is less than 1,300, then round up. If your number is more than 2,800, then round down to 2,800. If this number is higher than you are accustomed to, yet you have not been chronically dieting, then I suggest adding 50-100 calories per week, no more. Each subsequent week add 50-100 calories until you reach your target number. This way, you give the body a chance to adapt to the change and prevent any "freaking out" or rebound weight gain.

STEP 4:

Refer to the table below to determine the number of servings per food group that you may have each day. **From High Carb to Low Carb** or from **Low Carbohydrate Lifestyle, Already?** you know how many servings of fruit and complex carbohydrates you need to eat when you start the program. It is safe to start with two servings of fruit and between zero and two servings of complex carbohydrates. Print off a few pages of the **Meal and Serving Tracker** provided in the Resources menu at journeytowardjoy.com. Post this on your refrigerator or somewhere that you will use it, to keep track of your daily intake.

STEP 5:

Each day, keep track of your reactions to food with the **Food and Reaction Tracker** located in the resources menu of journeytowardjoy.com. Also, track your progress using the **Progress Tracker,** also provided in Resources menu at journeytowardjoy.com. Track your progress for two to three months.

STEP 6 (OPTIONAL):

If, and only if, you have completed this program for two to three months and you experience a considerable plateau (no changes in weight or measurements for three weeks), then feel free to play around with suggestions for your particular body type discussed in later chapters or review **Breaking through the Plateau.** Try one recommendation for a couple of weeks before you add another. This way you can gauge what works for your body. Once you see a shift, stick to this new change until you see improvements diminish, then try a new suggestion. DO NOT try multiple tips at once. Trying too many ideas at the same time puts undue stress on the body, and you will not know what is working and what is not working.

Let's Get Started

In the chart below you will find a suggested number of servings for each food group to have each day. Keep in mind; it is a range we are looking for and a weekly average, not a precise target number. The chart is meant to be a guide to keep you on track toward your goals. However, if you want precision and you like to track your food intake (I do from time to time to make sure I am getting all of my nutrients in), I suggest using a phone application like My Fitness Pal, or Cronometer to keep you focused. Also, once you feel comfortable with the meal planning and tracking of your servings, you can choose to tweak your plan using the suggested parameters provided for your somatotype (see chapter 10 for details). Otherwise, stick to these guidelines in this section and you will be well on your way to optimizing your nutrition and reaching your goals. Start with two servings of fruit and the amount of complex carbohydrate servings you have determined your body can tolerate (whether you are starting out low carb or high carb) but, no more than two servings. Your servings of protein can vary based upon your workout schedule or your hunger levels. Cheats are always optional and not necessary, depending upon your goals.

TIP:

Each "cheat" replaces one carbohydrate or fruit.
When choosing your complex carbohydrates stick to
*the **GREEN** choices in your approved food list. You*
*may feel free to try a **BLACK** item once per week.*
See recipes at the end of this book for more meal

*plan ideas. Also, check out the **Meal and Serving Tracker** for a blank version of the chart below, located in the Resources menu at* journeytowardjoy.-com, *to track your servings. The fruit, complex carbohydrates and cheats are optional for those who want to follow a very low carb lifestyle and wish to optimize their overall health.*

CALORIES	1,300-1,500	1,501-1,800	1,801-2,100	2,100-2,300	2,301-2,500	2,501-2,800
VEGETABLES	7-10	7-10	7-10	10	10	10
FRUITS	*2	*2	*2	*2	*2	*2
MEAT/ PROTEIN	3-4	3-4	4-5	4-5	5-6	5-6
COMPLEX CARBS	*0-2	*0-2	*0-2	*0-2	*0-2	*0-2
FATS	3	3	4	4	5	5
NUTS & SEEDS	1	1	2	2	3	3
OILS & BUTTERS	2	3	4	4	6	7
*CHEATS (replace one carb or fruit)	*0-2	*0-2	*0-2	*0-2	*0-2	*0-2

These items are entirely optional for you. Remember that one cheat replaces a serving of fruit or a complex carbohydrate.

For the sample meal plans below, I have included three meals, with two snacks. While snacking has been given a lot of criticism lately, the truth is that most stagnant weight loss can be traced back to hormone imbalance, adrenal stress and cortisol release. One of the best ways to keep your adrenals happy is to incorporate regular feeding times. If you suspect that your stress levels have contributed to your weight concerns, then please consider the following eating schedule:

1) Breakfast about an hour after waking and should include lots of protein, a serving of fruit and some vegetables.
2) 2-3 hours later have your first snack of either a vegetable and a protein or fruit and a protein

3) Lunch should consist of an approved protein, fat and lots of vegetables.

4) 2-3 hours later have your second snack of either a fruit and protein or a protein smoothie with fruit.

5) Dinner should be eaten before 7 pm to ensure that all digestion completes before bedtime. Dinner should consist of approved protein, fat, lots of vegetables.

6) Optional: If your body can process complex carbohydrates, then have them either for breakfast or dinner.

7) Optional: Add in a cheat such as dark chocolate or red wine and substitute either a serving of fruit or complex carbohydrate.

Sample Meal Plan (1300-1500 Calories):

Breakfast

Cinnamon pancakes (with almond flour) topped with 1/2 TBL of Kerrygold® butter and cooked in 1/2 TBL of coconut oil
Kale and spinach smoothie made with 3/4 cups of blackberries

Snack

Granny Smith apple with 2 TBL of almond butter

Lunch

Ground beef chili topped with guacamole made from 1/4 a large avocado
2 cups of roasted broccoli made with 1/2 TBL of coconut oil, sea salt, pepper and coconut aminos

Dinner

Beef Lettuce Wraps

Evening snack

(optional) 1 oz of 85% dark chocolate

Sample Meal Plan (18001-2100 Calories):

Breakfast

Chocolate Berry Smoothie

Snack

Cucumber salad made with apple cider vinegar, sea salt pepper, sliced cherry tomatoes, and freshly chopped cilantro

Lunch

Buffalo chicken made with 2 TBL of Kerrygold® butter served over 2 cups of shredded cabbage, topped with 1-2 TBL of home-made guacamole from 1 whole avocado
1 oz serving of toasted nuts

Snack

Protein smoothie made with 3/4 cup of berries, almond milk, and protein powder.

Dinner

Salmon cakes

3 cups of roasted cauliflower mash topped with 1 TBL of Kerry-gold® butter

Evening snack

(optional) 5 oz of red wine

I have provided some snack ideas in the **Recipes** section of this book if you get stumped as to what choices you may have.

Ultimately, losing weight is not necessarily about calories in versus calories out. In essence, your metabolic rate is determined by the overall quality and quantity of your calories in a day. Metabolism has more to do with how well nourished your body is, your quality of sleep, your hormonal balance, your workout efficiency, etc. It is important to note that while I recommend that starting this by eating 4-5 times per day, there is always room for adjustments after you have attempted this plan for at least eight weeks.

Lately, in the diet industry, eating less often and frequent fasting is getting much praise. And, the truth is that periodic fasting is beneficial for you IF YOUR ADRENALS AREN'T HAGGARD. I find that almost every woman with weight issues has imbalanced cortisol. Therefore, not eating regularly, stresses the adrenal glands further. The result? The adrenals will cause the release of sugar into the blood stream from the liver. When cortisol spikes the pancreas secretes insulin. The combination of increased cortisol and insulin is the perfect recipe for increased fat accumulation and potential burning up of lean muscle.

Yes, it is true that eating often spikes your insulin levels. But how HIGH it spikes depends on the quality of your food and the level of blood glucose created from your food choices. Because our goal is to keep you in a fat burning mode all day and night long, we must keep the adrenal health in mind, first and foremost. However, after trying the program for eight weeks, if you find that there are issues with your hormone balance or you stop burning fat, then eating less often may be the option that works for *your* body. I'll walk you through the steps in this chapter. Keep in mind that eating less often does not mean you will eat fewer foods or fewer calories! On the contrary, you will be eating larger, more satisfying meals 3-4 times per day, depending on your preference.

> TIP:
> *See **Recipes** for more meal plan ideas. Also, go to journeytowardjoy.com for the printable version of your **Meal and Serving Tracker** in the Resources menu. Use this blank chart to track your servings of each food group, each day:*

Recognize the Hormonal Indicators that may Need Adjusting.

When determining if you should alter your current eating plan, you should be clear on where to start. Whether you have been eating a diet that is **Low Carbohydrate, Already?** Or you have been eating a diet that required following the **From High Carb to Low Carb** plan; you will start **The Plan** with having two servings of approved fruits. Unless you have determined that your body operates well with under 50 net grams of carbohydrates per day (grams of fiber subtracted from total carbs), then you will start with two servings of fruit. If you are not sure if your body responds to very low carbohydrate intake, then keep reading.

I will provide you all the necessary assessments to determine if you need to make adjustments in your macronutrients. In addition to fruit intake, you will have only the tolerated amount of complex carbohydrates (zero to two servings per day) that you discovered in the week by week plan outlined in **Low Carbohydrate, Already?** or **From High Carb to Low Carb**. Once you have determined the servings of fruit and carbohydrate servings you will have each day, then, you will plan on eating the prescribed amount of vegetables, fats and protein servings, based upon your caloric need. There are several rules of thumb to consider as you plan your meals each day. Also, there are several signs to look out for to determine if you need to make adjustments in your servings of your macronutrients (protein, fat, and carbohydrates).

Start with a minimum of three meals per day. Three meals per day allow your body to have time to burn fat in-between meals, yet it receives enough nutrient information to determine that food is not scarce and famine is not an issue. As you go through your day, pay close attention to the signals your body may provide that point to the need for further tweaking of your plan. Every day you should be tracking your food (in the beginning) and your body's reaction to your choice in meals. You can track these symptoms using the

Meal and Reaction Tracker from the resource tab at journeyto-wardjoy.com.

How do you know if you are on track toward balancing your hormones? How can you tell if you need to make adjustments? What modifications can you make? These are all excellent questions that deserve answers. In this next section, I'll dive into the hormonal indicators that you are indeed on track. Dr. Jade Teta, N.D., and Dr. Keoni Teta, N.D., founders of The Metabolic Effect (www.metaboliceffect.com) and authors of *Lose Weight Here* provide three leading indicators to watch for: hunger energy and cravings (HEC). I suggest you refer to their books for more about how to conquer these roadblocks. For this book, I have included some additional indicators based on my clinical observations, which are either common complaints associated with the inability to lose weight or demonstrated through laboratory testing. The primary indicators I will focus on in this book include sleep, hunger, energy, cravings, digestion, mood and exercise performance.

Here are the questions you will need to ask yourself each day:

Did I sleep soundly and wake to feel rested?
Did I feel hungry in between my meals?
Did my energy crash at any point today? What time did this occur?
Did I have cravings for food that does not benefit me (i.e., too much coffee, sugar, fat, salt)?

Did I have digestive issues after I ate a meal (bloating, gas, cramping, etc.)

Did I suffer from mood changes throughout the day?

Did my performance suffer during my workout, today?

If you answered "yes" to any of these questions, then you will need to investigate a bit further. It is most likely that you are experiencing an imbalance in the favorable hormonal pathways that lead to fat loss. Let's dig a bit deeper into each of these questions so that you can tailor your regimen, accordingly.

SLEEP

If your sleep was affected, then rule out some of the common causes. If you drank alcohol the night before, consider giving it a break for a while. Did you have caffeine later in the day than usual? You may need to try cutting down on your caffeine intake. Did you have too many liquids before your bed time and the urgency to urinate is getting you out of bed? Try stopping your liquid intake three hours before bedtime. Are you struggling with mind racing thoughts? Try journaling before bed, making a list of "to-do's" for the next day, and listening to a guided meditation for sleep once you hit the pillow at night. Did you wake up often at night for no reason? You may need to have your cortisol levels tested and ask your holistic practitioner for assistance in managing cortisol at night. Other ways to help you sleep include analyzing your last meal before bed. If it was low in protein and fat, then increase these first. Otherwise, try adding in carbohydrates to your dinner and pay attention to your body's reactions.

INCREASED HUNGER

If you are hungry between meals, then mismanagement of your leptin and insulin levels is likely. Was your hunger a real growling of your stomach or was it a mental desire to eat food? If it is the latter, ask yourself if there is a reward that you are seeking from the food? Can you provide the reward you seek from a non-food source? Try the non-food source method or drink two large glasses of water. If you are hungry between meals, first increase your water intake between meals. Then, if you are still hungry, and you are unable to make it four to five hours between meals, then you know you need to adjust your meals. After increasing water intake, then increase the ounces of protein and increase fibrous vegetables. If you are having four ounces of protein at a meal, try six ounces or eight ounces. If you have lettuce for lunch, try having broccoli instead. If you are still hungry, add one tablespoon of fat to your meal. If you are still struggling with hunger, then add in one serving of complex carbohydrate. Lastly, if all of the above fail to improve your hunger symptoms, add in a snack of protein and vegetables so that you are having four or five meals, instead of three.

DECREASED ENERGY

There are many possible reasons for reduced energy. First, make sure your sleep is properly managed and carry out the necessary adjustments as described above. If you aren't sleeping well, then it is possible that cortisol and insulin imbalance are to blame. First, assess your stress levels. Are you managing your stress appropriately? If not, see the help for stress reduction providing in **Break-**

ing through the Plateau. Are you drinking too much coffee? Titrate your intake down to no more than one-half a cup to one cup of caffeinated beverages per day. What time of day did your energy crash? Were you properly hydrated? If not, have two glasses of water. Did you workout today? If so, was the workout too intense? If so, you'll need to tone it down until you know your body's sweet spot for maintaining energy. Then, take a look at the meal you had just before the crash. You may want to try adding in more protein to this meal. If you are still feeling fatigued, add in a serving of fat or carbohydrate, based upon what was low in this meal, and see if your energy improves. Lastly, if these options do not increase your energy, try adding a snack during this time.

CRAVINGS

The cause(s) of cravings can be very complex. Usually, cravings involve an increase in stress hormones (such as cortisol), or diminished neurotransmitter function (such as dopamine and serotonin) or a combination of both. Stress is a key component when unlocking the mystery to cravings as well. You see, stress increases the release of cortisol and increases the activity of the reward centers (dopamine). The increase in both cortisol and reward centers create the perfect storm for shutting down the more "reasonable" aspects of the brain causing you to feel less motivated and more likely to pounce on food in a primitive nature. You will feel more inclined to attack the nearest salty, sugary, fatty food. Thus, in combination, dopamine (desire) and cortisol (stress) create a recipe for disaster: "need and want" combined with "must have it now." Also, cravings can be a sign of deficiency in nutrients. For example, a craving for chocolate can be the body's need for magnesium as cacao is one of the highest sources. The key with cravings is to determine if there is a mental, emotional component that must be ruled out, first. Is there something that you are longing for that a particular food provides. Is it comfort? Is it relaxation? Is it a sense of euphoria? How about the need for indulgence and an "I deserve a reward" mentality? Address these longings with non-food methods first. Try coffee with a girlfriend; binge-watch your favorite comedy show; take a hot bath and sip on tea; attend your favorite yoga class, etc.

If you are feeling stressed, take the time to practice deep breathing, go for a gentle walk and have some tea that is high in calming properties (both Yogi Tea and Traditional Medicinals Tea companies have great stress-relieving teas). If you have ruled out an emotional component to your cravings and stress is under control, then assess if you have signs of low blood sugar. An excellent way to determine this is to eat a snack. If you eat a green apple and two hard-boiled eggs and feel back to normal, then most likely your previous meal was not large enough, your workouts are too intense, you are sleep deprived, or you need to add in a snack. You'll have to play around with your routine to get to the bottom of what *your* body is telling you.

DIGESTIVE ISSUES

Digestive issues can be caused by food sensitivities, intestinal inflammation leading to gut lining permeability, inadequate digestive enzymes, inadequate fiber intake, etc. Signs and symptoms that may indicate you have digestive issues include gas, bloating, stomach pain, and changes in bowel habits. For most people, the onset of discomfort is rather immediate (within a couple of hours of the last meal). Keep track of your food intake and your body's response to the foods using the Meal and Reaction tracker located on the Resources tab at journeytowardjoy.com. A good rule of thumb is to eliminate common allergens such as grains, dairy, eggs, soy, beans (including peanuts), potatoes, tomatoes, and peppers. Of course, you have eliminated sugar as this can wreak havoc on your gut biome (or flora). In general, you'll only be eating clean protein sources, vegetables, fruits, nuts (except peanuts), seeds and non-dairy fats. Follow this uncomplicated eating plan for two weeks to one month. Then, every three days, reintroduce ONE food type at a time to your diet and gauge how you feel.

TIP:

I highly encourage you to seek professional help for testing food sensitivities; but if you are low on cash, the method as mentioned earlier is a simple way to determine if you are sensitive to the significant players. I suggest that when reintroducing a food group that you take your pulse, first. Wait ten minutes after introducing the food and retake your pulse. If your pulse elevates ten beats per minute or more, you are more than likely suffering from a reaction to that food.

I highly recommend that after you have eliminated these foods for a month or so, that you invest in a quality digestive enzyme supplement, a probiotic from a trusted company and that you rebuild the gut lining and repair any "holes" and permeability caused by inflammatory foods. An inexpensive way to do this is to have homemade bone broth three times per day. You can also invest in a product designed for this that includes L-glutamine. Other ingredients that are helpful are aloe, licorice root, and brush border enzymes. Most people will benefit from following this or a similar protocol a few times a year to re-establish healthy gut function.

MOOD CHANGES:

So many variables affect mood. Not getting enough sleep, not eating enough food, and not exercising or exercising too much can impact mood. Granted, it is always wise to test your neurotransmitter function if you suspect your attitude change is a result of neurotransmitter imbalance. If the disposition change is more sudden, more temporary and seems to fluctuate with the change in habits, then the issue more likely lies in the former (sleep, food or exercise) than the latter (neurotransmitter function). If you suspect that food is the issue, try eating more frequently, especially if you think low blood sugar is an issue. If you lack in sleep, follow the protocols suggested in this book outlined in **Preparing For Success**, to assist in enhancing sleep. If you are eating lower carbohydrate content, try adding in one serving to one meal. Make sure your protein intake is adequate and appropriate for your body weight (0.75-1.0 grams per pound of body weight is safe). Protein chains contain amino acids, and amino acids are the building blocks to neurotransmitters responsible for contentment and satisfaction. Feel free to add in branched chain amino acids (BCAAs) to your daily routine as well. The health benefits are extensive. If you are experiencing anxiety, make sure you address these concerns with your practitioner, in addition to addressing your stress levels appropriately. For tips check out the **Breaking through the Plateau** portion of this book.

EXERCISE PERFORMANCE:

You'll know if your exercise performance starts to suffer. What used to be a workout that made your stronger over time, is now causing you to feel weak and unable to meet the required demands to maintain proper form, alignment, and completion of each movement. If your performance starts to suffer, this is a huge sign that you are underfeeding your body or you are over-training. Try adding in a serving of complex carbohydrates after your workout and at dinner (if you work out in the morning). Make sure that you are eating enough throughout the day. If your hunger is increasing and your energy is decreasing, you have not hit the "sweet spot" of nutrition or exercise balance. Take a hard look at your training. If you are attending a cross fit class four times a week and running on the weekends, you most likely are burning precious fuel. Dial down your workouts to the bare minimum until your nutrition is in check and then make adjustments based upon your activity level. For example, on an HIIT day or circuit training day, I will eat four times a day and add in two servings of sweet potato. On yoga, walking or hiking day, I'll eat three times a day and have only one serving of sweet potato and limit my fruit and fats. It is essentially a method of maximizing hormonal response to food and exercise to get the results you want.

Making Adjustments to Your Nutrition if any of the Above Indicators of Imbalance are Present

If you answered "yes" to any of the questions listed above,(sleep, hunger, decreased energy, food cravings, sleep disturbances, mood changes, digestive issues and exercise performance) then your plan will require some tweaking. Some adjustments may not be food related at all. If you suspect this, I have provided both food and non-food adjustments that you can try as aforementioned above. If you have tried the non-food adjustments and need a clear cut approach toward addressing your food, then I suggest you follow the method outlined for you below. Keep in mind that you will need to address each one, in the order provided, trying only *one* option at a time. Try each method for two to three days, with no other changes, and look for any improvements in your noted imbalances. *Note: once you start to experience balance and you see improvement, then you need not progress any further as you have solved the issue.* Make the necessary adjustments to your Food Tracking (i.e., the suggested servings of each food group), and you now have your plan that promotes balance and turns up fat burning mechanisms. Here are the steps, in the order that you will try, for continual fat loss:

1) Increase water intake first to make sure the body is properly hydrated (at least half your body weight in ounces of water per day). Ideally, you will work up to drinking your body weight in ounces of water, each day.

2) Add more protein and green fibrous veggies to each meal. You can start with adding a serving of each, per day.

3) Add in a serving of fat, starting with one tablespoon of coconut oil.

4) Add in one complex carbohydrate serving per day. The best time to have this complex carbohydrate is right after strength training or intense exercise. If you are not exercising intensely, then have the starch in the morning or at night; but not at lunch.

5) Take out one serving of fat or one serving of carbohydrate.

6) Add in a snack consisting of protein and fibrous vegetables.

7) Don't forget that if cravings are an issue, then let yourself have an approved "cheat." If it means keeping you on track by allowing a treat now and then, then it is better not to feel deprived.

I suggest that you follow the caloric and serving suggestions in this chapter for two to three months and track your progress using the **Daily and Weekly Trackers** located in the Resource menu at journeytowardjoy.com. If at any time you notice that you are no longer losing weight or inches, then you can look to suggested changes for your body type or the plateau-breaking suggestions listed later in this book. As a rule of thumb, if you have tried The

Plan for two to three months and your fat loss stalls, your measurements are no longer improving, or you are gaining weight, you can customize your program further.

What if I am Hormonally Balanced (no Indicators Present), but I am no Longer Losing Fat?

If your sleep, hunger, energy cravings, digestion, mood and physical performance are balanced and you do not see substantial progress toward your physical goals, then adjustments in your food may be necessary. ALWAYS MAKE CHANGES IN THE KITCHEN FIRST! In other words: it is most likely that your workouts are *not* the problem.

It should be stated again, for the record that before you change your suggested servings of **The Plan**, you should give it at least two full months before you determine that change is necessary. Two months allows your body the required time to adapt—and to catch up to, the change. If your measurements have changed for the better, but the scale has not budged, then keep doing what you are doing: It is working! The scale doesn't distinguish between weight gained in lean muscle mass or water weight. For each of the suggestions below, try ONE at a time, for *one to two weeks* BEFORE moving to the next step. If you see success, you do not need to progress to the next stage. You have found the solution. Here are the steps so that you will try them for continual fat loss:

1) Double check your caloric intake. Track your intake on My Fitness Pal or Cronometer for three days. For this step, you don't need a full week to figure out your daily caloric intake. Are you in range? Move to step two.
2) Cut back on your starches, alcohol and "legal cheats."
3) Move all your complex carbohydrates to one meal (ideally post workout or at dinner)
4) Take out a serving or two of fat.
5) If you are eating snacks, try going back to three meals.
6) On cardio days (yoga, walking, dancing, etc.) to having only three main meals, zero to one snack and zero to one serving of complex carbohydrate. On your cardio days have a lower fat intake as well. On days that you perform HIIT training or circuit training, have three meals, two snacks and two servings of complex carbohydrate (one after your workout, one at dinner).
7) Play with your snacks. If you are already snacking regularly, move back to three meals per day. If you are eating three meals per day, try adding one snack during the day (especially on days you do weight training or intense exercise).

There is no one-size-fits-all approach to fat loss. As you can see, the fat loss plan must be tailor-made for your body (including your hormonal landscape and your metabolism). The guidelines that I have provided you will be paramount in monitoring your progress and making the necessary adjustments.

Let's summarize how to make alterations to *your* eating plan:

1) If you have tried **The Plan** for two months and you no longer see progress, then ensure that your hormonal indicators are balanced (sleep, hunger, energy, cravings, digestion, mood and physical performance). First, follow the non-food suggestions provided. If you try the non-food recommendations and your hormone indicators are still not balanced or optimized, then make the necessary food-related adjustments by following steps one through seven, starting with increasing your water intake.

2) If all indicators are stable and you are struggling with your progress toward fat loss, then follow steps one through seven to aid in a further fat loss, starting with double-checking your caloric intake.

3) If your indicators of hormone imbalance are in check and you have tried each step for continual fat burning, and you need further assistance, then you may choose to dive even deeper into the world of customization. Feel free to read more suggestions outlined in **Calculating Your Macronutrient Intake for Your Body Type**. You may choose to follow the "Simpler Suggestion" for each of the body types discussed in later chapters or, if you are more "Type A" in your eating habits, you can choose to follow precise calculations and tracking methods to create specific meal plans based upon your goal. A hint for you: start with nutrition first. Again, it is my recommendation that you do not attempt adjustments until you have a handle on the ap-

propriate caloric intake and serving sizes outlined in this chapter. Do I sound like a broken record, yet?

4) Lastly, if you have tried all of the suggested methods for continued fat loss outlined in this chapter or you decide to try suggestions for your body type (in later chapters), and your progress comes to a halt, then take a look at the tips provided in **Breaking through the Plateau.**

The goal is to help you to make appropriate adjustments as *you* deem necessary. *No clear cut path works for everyone* when it comes to health and fitness. The process must be viewed as an experiment as you find what works best for you and your body type.

In the next chapter, I'll discuss a simpler way of addressing fitness. The good news? You don't have to work out longer to obtain the results you are seeking. The contrary is true. Science has proven that shorter bouts of high-intensity work and lower intensity cardio combined with strength training can provide incredible results that will shift your body composition in a more favorable direction.

Chapter 10

The Plan: Creating Your Workout Routine

Improve Your Body Composition Using Proven Methods that are Effective and Efficient!

Creating a physique that is the range of optimal Body Mass Index, body fat, lean muscle tissue, etc. doesn't have to be a complicated process. The goal is obviously to decrease the size of fat tissue and to increase the amount of lean body mass. Believe it or not, most of your fat burning (approximately 70-80%) is possible with eating a balanced, whole food, nutritionally dense, portion-controlled diet. Yep! That's it. You do not need to run on a treadmill or an elliptical for an hour a day to burn fat. In fact, the repetitive motion of chronic cardiovascular exercise can damage your joints and waste lean muscle tissue. Furthermore, you can achieve your ideal physique with a lot less effort than you think! Sounds too good to be true, right? Take a look at the people who attend your Zumba class each week or the folks in your spin class. If you've been at the fitness center long enough, you've probably noticed that most physiques have not changed much, if at all. Is it a waste of time? Well, not entirely; but, if you could work out less with better results, wouldn't you do it?

So, what type of exercise should you be doing? I suggest that you pick some light to moderately intense (and fun) cardiovascular exercises that bring you joy and do these for 2-3 hours per week. Pick something that is not intense but will get your heart rate up, and you can have a conversation during your workout if needed. For example, a 1-hour hike one day, a 1-hour yoga class another day, a 45-minute dance class another day, etc. My personal favorite to do each day for 10-20 minutes: jumping on a mini trampoline! You can do this while watching your favorite TV program. 20 minutes per day will add up to a little over two hours in a week. And, as a bonus to the fun, the health benefits of a mini trampoline are endless.

Next, you will need to increase lean muscle tissue by doing all over body resistance training. You can lift weights, or you can do my favorite: calisthenic training using your body weight. Do a form of resistance training for the entire body twice a week for 30-45 minutes. For beginners, I suggest checking out Mark Lauren's You Are Your Own Gym Beginner workout on YouTube. You can get an entire body workout in less than 20 minutes. If you prefer, you can choose some of the most tried and true body resistance exercises and do a set of each and repeat the entire set three to four times. For example:

1) The most pushups you can do at once (keep your spine straight, bottom down and eyes slightly in front of you. Try hands close together, wide apart, etc. to change it up. Start on your

knees or against a wall if you aren't quite strong enough for a full-body push up. But don't be discouraged. Your strength will improve. Alternate this exercise with pull up exercises, such as chin ups using a bar or a modified version with a chin up bar while standing on a chair and using as much of your body weight as you can. If this is too much, you can try using a sturdy kitchen countertop or table, lying on the ground face up, palms facing toward your face and gripping the countertop or table above you, then pulling your body weight upward. You can try straight or bent knees, depending on your strength level.

2) Alternate lunge exercises, each leg 30 times. Never push your knee more forward than your ankle and keep your pelvis tucked in and your back kept straight. If you want to add more resistance, hold dumbbells.

3) Hold a plank for as long as you are able. Start with 30 seconds and work up to 2 minutes. Start on your elbows and your knees, if you need to. Alternate this exercise with swimmer exercises. For the swimmer's exercise, lie on your abdomen palms facing down and arms straight above your head. Extend your arms (keep them

straight) and your legs. Lift your head, arms, and legs above the ground. Use a kicking motion with your feet and an up and down motion with your arms to create a "swimming-like" motion. Do this for 30 seconds to start and work up to 2 minutes.

4) Sumo squats x 30. Make sure to point your toes slightly out, feet a little wider than hips width, bend at the hips and let your bottom drop to just below knee level. Make sure that the knees are directly over your heel and the back is straight. Make sure to squeeze your glutes as you straighten your body. To add to the intensity lift your toes a bit and add dumbbells.

Repeat the above round three to four times. Make sure to work each muscle group to fatigue and failure (you cannot do another repetition). Working a muscle group to failure is how you break down the muscle so it can rebuild and become stronger (and you become leaner). If you did not fatigue a muscle group at the end of a set, you need more resistance. Try adding weights, increasing your repetitions, increasing your number of rounds or all three. The goal is to fatigue the muscle group and to feel that you maintained an effort level of 7-8 on a scale of 1-10 throughout your rounds.

Lastly, to turn up the fat loss, incorporate at least one day of High-Intensity Interval Training (HIIT). HIIT will boost fat burning for

24-48 hours post workout. The best part? You only need to do it for 4-15 minutes.

There are many ways to do HIIT training. One of the easiest ways is sprinting; however, if you have joint pain or musculoskeletal issues that prevent such intensity, you can "sprint" using a stationary bike, a jump rope, a mini trampoline, etc. Here is one routine that I like:

Warm up with a brisk walk or an easy ride for 3-5 minutes. Once your muscles are warm, perform the following:

1) Go at a moderate pace (around a 6-7 on exertion scale of 1-10) for 30 seconds.
2) Then go as fast you possibly can (9-10 on exertion scale) for 10-15 seconds.
3) Recover by moving at an easy pace (around 2 or 3 on exertion scale) for 1 minute.

Repeat this cycle 4-10 times, depending on your ability. If your goal is to step up the fat burning, try incorporating your HIIT twice a week (or even three); however, never on days that are back to back and never if you are feeling fatigued or if you did not achieve adequate sleep, the evening before your workout.

TIP:
See the menu Resources at journeytowardjoy.com *for a customizable, printable **Workout Planner.** You*

can use the sample month of workouts on the fol-
lowing page.

Sample Month of Workouts:

	SUN	MON	TUE	WED	THU	FRI	SAT
WEEK 1	2 hour hike	30 minutes body weight training	30 minutes yoga; 20 minutes HIIT	30 minutes body weight training	1 hour walk	30 minutes yoga; 20 minutes HIIT	REST
WEEK 2	1 hour walk	30 minutes body weight training	15 minutes HIIT	1 hour walk	30 minutes body weight training	30 minutes yoga; 15 minutes HIIT	REST
WEEK 3	REST	10 minutes HIIT; 1 hour walk	30 minutes yoga	45 minutes body weight training	15 minutes HIIT	30 minutes body weight training	2 hour hike
WEEK 4	REST	45 minutes body weight training	1 hour hike	15 minutes HIIT; 30 minutes yoga	30 minutes body weight training	1 hour walk	15 minutes HIIT; 30 minutes yoga

Up to this point, you have learned the importance of changing your mindset and clearing out or de-cluttering the untrue thoughts that prevent you from moving toward your goals. You now know what foods to focus on for optimizing your nutrition. You know how to look for indicators that your hormonal pathways are either moving toward fat loss or away from it. You can now make necessary adjustments to these indicators as well as how to tweak your macronutrients for continued fat loss. Lastly, in this chapter, you have obtained the tools required for creating an exercise plan to strengthen, stretch and transform your body.

In the next chapter, I will share with you some valuable information that can help you fine-tune your nutrition based on your body type. Don't forget; it is best to try the prescribed method first for a couple of months to get a handle on the specified serving suggestions, your fitness, etc. If after that time you feel you need to make additional adjustments, you can start with **Determining Your Body Type** and **Calculate Your Macronutrient Intake for Your Body Type**, if you haven't seen the progress you desire. Otherwise, if you have seen progress, but you are at a plateau of three weeks or longer, then jump to **Breaking through the Plateau**.

PART 3
TAILORING YOUR PROGRAM

Chapter 11

Determining Your Body Type

Somatotype Explained

Now the above nutrition plan is great if you need something simple that applies to most people and is an easy method for moving in the direction for better health. However, if you wish to take the process a bit further and customize your eating and your workouts to fit your individualized body type, then it is necessary to introduce the three somatotypes: ectomorph, mesomorph, and endomorph. Some folks may find that they are a combination of somatotypes; however, what usually happens is they are the heavier version of one or the other and are mistaking themselves for the wrong type. Does this sound confusing? Don't worry. We'll work through the process of determining your type, together.

The best place to start is to think of your body in its best shape or when you were "in your prime." What did you look like before you started gaining weight or after you have lost weight in the past? This picture can help you when answering the questions regarding your body type.

You can take the overly simplified quiz I have created for you below, or you can use the quiz provided on this web page: http://www.bodybuilding.com/fun/becker3.htm

Somatotype Quiz

Are your shoulders:

    a)   the same width as your hips

    b)   wider than your hips

    c)   smaller than your hips

Regarding your weight, is it:

    a)   difficult to gain weight, but if I do it is in my belly primarily

    b)   easy to gain weight and lose weight with effort

    c)   impossible to lose weight even if I do all of the right things

My body shape when I am in my best shape is:

    a)   straight up and down, skinny

    b)   more athletic with defined musculature and a defined waist, hourglass; stay lean and muscular (men)

    c)   more pear-shaped, with more fat accumulation in the hips and thighs; carry a bit of extra fat (men)

When encircling my middle finger and thumb around my wrist:

    a)   my finger and thumb overlap

    b)   my finger and thumb touch

c) my finger and thumb do not touch

My chest measurements are:
a) 35 inches or less (female); 37 inches or less (male)
b) 35-42 inches (female); 37-42 inches (male)
c) 42 inches or more (female); 43 inches or more (male)

My forearms look:
a) small
b) average
c) big

My body appears:
a) long, thin and narrow
b) square or athletic
c) soft and rounder in parts

If you answered mostly "a" to the questions above, then you are most likely an **ectomorph**.
If you answered mostly "b," then you are most likely a **mesomorph**.
If you answered mostly "c," then you are most likely an **endomorph**.

Now that you have an idea of your body type, you can follow the food and fitness recommendations for your particular somatotype. If you are still unsure of your body type, I have provided some more specific characteristics of each to help you further define your somatotype.

Consider that you may be a combination of more than one body type. If this is the case, determine which type with which you mostly match. You can use a picture of your body at its best or a picture of you as a youth to determine your overall bone structure and appearance if this helps. The goal is to consider your inherited body type based on your skeletal frame and body composition.

Remember, that an overweight ectomorph or mesomorph may appear to be like an endomorph so keep in mind that just because you have some extra weight you are holding on to, this does not automatically mean you are an endomorph somatotype. Classic combinations may include an ecto-endomorph: an overweight ectomorph with a belly pouch and extra fat storage in the hips and thighs, but they maintain their thin, delicate upper bodies. Likewise, you can have an endo-ectomorph with higher fat storage in the mid section (apple shape) and small lower bodies like the ectomorph. Therefore, keep in mind that in these scenarios you will want to stick to that which is more dominant for a starting point.

Another way of assisting you in determining your body type is to eat your maintenance calories identified in **The Plan: Calculate Your Caloric Needs**; the amount you eat to maintain your weight. If you eat this for a week and you gain weight, you may be endomorph.

Use the below characteristics to guide you.

Ectomorph:

Small shoulders

Small chest

Tall, lean with little body fat and little muscle (think fashion model or basketball

player)

Can't gain weight easily

Small bone structure (middle finger and thumb overlap wrist bone)

Long legs and arms

Minimal fat storage

Less muscle mass

High metabolism

Difficulty gaining weight

Skinny

Narrow hips, waist, and clavicles

Stringy muscle bellies

Can gain weight in belly

Body has a flat look, including flatter backside

Can tend to be more naturally restrained in movement and intro-verted in social

situations (a stereotype so don't use this as a huge indicator)

Mesomorph:

Medium size bone structure (middle finger and thumb touch when wrapped around wrist bone)

Athletic build and strong

High metabolism

Easier to gain muscle and maintains muscle well

Gains fat easily

Rectangular shape

Broad shoulders line up with hips or may be wider than hips (upside down triangle)

Muscular, fit

Weight fluctuates a lot

Wide clavicles

Narrow waist

Thinner joints

Long and round muscle bellies

Can be more courageous, assertive and adventurous (a stereotype so don't use this as
a huge indicator)

Endomorph:

Softer, rounder look (think football lineman, Oprah Winfrey)

Do not have to be overweight to be this body type (think Marilyn Monroe or Kim Kardashian)

Large bone structure (middle finger and thumb do not touch when encircling wrist
bone)

More body mass with more body fat and underdeveloped muscle

Slow metabolism

Gains fat (and weight) quickly, harder to lose weight

Robust and muscular but you can't see it

Shorter stature

Pear-shaped, fat in lower region

Blocky

Thick rib cage

Full, thicker joints

Hips as wide or wider than shoulders

Shorter limbs

Big appetite

Can have slow reactions, disposed to more complacent behavior and enjoy food,

people, social events, and affection (a stereotype so don't use this as a huge indicator)

At this time, you should have a decent idea as to what somatotype you are; therefore, you can make better decisions when faced with food and fitness choices. In the next chapter, we will dive into some details about choosing the right amounts of carbohydrate, fats, and protein for your body type. Keep in mind that this chapter is not necessary for your nutritional success on this program. However, you may find it useful for tweaking your caloric intake or your suggested servings in the case that you have tried the prescribed nutrition guidelines for two months or more and your results aren't as favorable as you like. The next chapter is an additional tool for you to reference when determining pathways in your health and fitness journey.

Chapter 12

Calculating Your Macronutrient Intake for Your Body Type

A Method for Tracking Nutrition for the "Type A" Folks Who Need Even More Structure

For many of you, calculating your macronutrients (carbohydrates, fats, and protein) is far too much work. And for you, I suggest that you follow the portion-controlled serving approach as outlined in **The Plan: Calculate Your Caloric Needs**. Frankly, the portion-controlled approach is my preferred way to monitor my eating. I find calculating macronutrients to be very tiresome and to require far too much diligence. If you are more like me and you wish to keep things as simple as possible, then feel free to skip this chapter altogether, or you can review the "Simpler Suggestions" as a method to help you tailor your portion-controlled approach; to hone in on your individual needs.

Therefore, as a method of assisting those who do not wish to follow a macronutrient calculation but are interested in tailoring their portion-controlled approach to their body type, I recommend the "simpler" method (*). You will find the simpler method located below each of the macronutrient percentages provided for each body type. With the simpler method, you skip the macro nutrient calculations and formulations. I highly recommend that you use a phone app to help you calculate your macronutrient profile (My Fitness Pal). Using a phone app is an easy way to "check in" from time to time and to monitor your eating habits. By checking in once and a while, you can assess any hindrance in achieving your goals.

For those of you out there who wish to take a more controlled, calculative approach to your weight loss, I've included a more precise method for you. For starters in creating your macronutrient plan, review the suggested percentages and ranges provided below for your somatotype. When deciding whether to go with the lower end of the range or the higher end of range here are some helpful hints to assist you: In general, if you have a lot of weight to lose, a lower carbohydrate intake and higher fat intake will benefit you. If you are close to your weight loss goal or you have noticed that your energy, sleep, and workouts are suffering after two months of trying **The Plan**, then you may want to add in complex carbohydrates slowly and fruit and see if your weight shifts. As you adjust your carb intake up, you may need to adjust your fat intake down. Make sure that you make only one adjustment at a time and allow your body to adjust for a week or two. If you don't see improvements, then add in another adjustment.

Ectomorph Macronutrient Suggestions:

- 20-40% carbohydrate (from complex carbs, fruits, and vegetables)
- 30-50% fat
- 30% protein

Simpler Suggestion For the Ectomorph:

First make sure that you have addressed all indicators that your hormones are not balanced (i.e., sleep, hunger, energy, cravings, digestion, mood, fitness performance). Go back to **The Plan** and review how to address these areas, according to your imbalance.

You may be the body type that benefits from more complex carbohydrates; therefore, the suggested two servings may be perfect for you. Make sure you slowly add carbs in by following the suggestions in **Low Carbohydrate Lifestyle, Already?** to safely integrate carbohydrates into your diet, especially if you have been eating lower carb levels for a while. With this method, you will have more control over how your body responds, and you can make the necessary adjustments. Make sure to monitor your reactions (i.e., gas, bloating, etc.) as discussed in **The Plan: Calculate Your Caloric Needs.** If you experience any negative symptoms, then eliminate that food group for now or reduce the serving sizes a bit.

Once you figure out the safe amount of complex carbohydrates for your body (zero to two servings), try
this number of servings for a week. If things start to
budge, then stay with this plan.

Then, if your weight isn't budging, try moving all of
your carbohydrates to one meal (ideally after a workout, in the am or at dinner). Do this for one week. If
things are moving in a favorable direction, stay here.
If your weight still is not budging, try taking out a
serving or two of fat. Try this for one week. If things
are moving and shaking, then stay here.

You can also try to change up your eating based on
your workouts. On cardio days (yoga, walking, dancing, etc.) have only three meals and zero to one serving of complex carbohydrate. On these days have a
lower fat intake as well. On days that you have HIIT
training or circuit training, have four meals with two
servings of complex carbohydrate (one after your
workout, one at dinner). Again, if things are working
after a week, stay here.

Otherwise, Play with your snacks. If you currently
incorporate snacks, you can play with scaling back to
three meals per day. If you are eating three meals per

day, try adding one snack during the day (especially on days you do weight training or intense exercise).

Mesomorph Macronutrient Suggestions:

- 20-30% carbohydrate
- 30-40% fat
- 30-40% protein
- Stop eating when you feel 75% full.
- Watch your calorie intake regularly with Google, My Fitness Pal or Cronometer.

Simpler Suggestion for the Mesomorph:

Stick to the outline given to you in **The Plan: Calculate Your Caloric Needs** for your total servings of carbohydrates, fat, and protein. As you get closer to your goal or your activity levels change, you may need to make some adjustments. It is necessary to make subtle adjustments to see how your body reacts as your body type is *very* sensitive to macronutrient changes and responds rather quickly.

First make sure that you have addressed all indicators that your hormones are not balanced (i.e., sleep, hunger, energy, cravings, digestion, mood, fitness performance).

Go back to **The Plan** and review how to address these areas, according to your imbalance.

Once you address any indicators of imbalance, then check your caloric intake. Track it for three days to make sure you are "in range." If not, carry out the necessary adjustments. If after a week your body shape and measurements start to change, you are in the right zone. Stay here.

If you are not moving in a favorable direction by the end of a week, try increasing your protein (between 0.8-1.0 gram per pound of lean body mass) and fibrous vegetable servings by one and decrease your complex carbohydrate intake by one serving. Cut alcohol down to one day per week, if you haven't done so already. If things start to budge, then stay with this plan.

Then, if your weight isn't budging, try moving all of your carbohydrates to one meal (ideally after a workout, in the am or at dinner). Do this for one week. If things are moving in a favorable direction, stay here. If your weight still is not budging, try taking out a serving or two of fat. Try this for one week. If things are moving and shaking, then stay here.

If you don't see progress, then cut back on your fat intake by one to two servings. If progress occurs, stay here. If not, continue to the next option after a week.

You can also try to change up your eating based on your workouts. On cardio days (yoga, walking, dancing, etc.) have only three meals and zero to one serving of complex carbohydrate. On these days have a lower fat intake as well. On days that you have HIIT training or circuit training, have four meals with two servings of complex carbohydrate (one after your workout, one at dinner). Again, if things are working after a week, stay here. If your workouts are suffering, you are feeling fatigued throughout the day, or your sleep starts to suffer, then you may need to slowly add in a fruit or a carbohydrate serving, up to 30% of your total intake.

Otherwise, play with your snacks. If you snack between meals, try eating three meals per day. If you are eating three meals per day, try adding one snack during the day (especially on days you do weight training or intense exercise).

It is vital for you to monitor your macros with your phone app so that you can make sure you are meeting these requirements each day. Even if every meal isn't perfect, you can shoot for staying within the "window" by either using a phone app or following the serving suggestions in **The Plan: Calculate Your Caloric Needs.** Pay attention to your body as the mesomorph body type responds the quickest to slight adjustments. Make sure you make *one* change at a time. With every change, you should give yourself a week or two to see if the scale budges or if your measurements decrease. In this manner, you can play around a bit to see how your own body reacts to the increasing or decreasing macronutrient profiles. You will need to measure your food, regardless, to stay within these guidelines. If you are moving in the right direction, stick to the new plan.

It is a matter of playing around with your servings to find the "sweet spot." As long as you are tracking your response to food each day and journaling each day: your digestion, your sleep, your energy levels, and your hunger, etc. you can get a good idea as to whether or not you body is responding well to your plan. **Use the Daily Tracker** or **Weekly Tracker** found under the menu "Resources" at journeytowardjoy.com.

Endomorph Macronutrient Suggestions:

- 5-15% carbohydrate for fat loss
- 60-70% fat
- 25-30% protein

- Watch your carbohydrate intake (if you have more weight to lose, keep your carbohydrates lower).
- I suggest that you have a lower fruit intake of zero to one serving per day, no more.
- Eat protein at each meal.
- When eating yogurt, avoid any low fat or non-fat versions.
- Increase your carbohydrate intake with vegetables only.
- Allow yourself weekly scheduled cheats (1-3x per week)
- Avoid complex carbohydrate (until you reach your goal) and get carbohydrates from vegetables.

Simpler Suggestion for the Endomorph:

First, make sure that you have preemptively addressed all suspected indicators of hormones imbalance (i.e., sleep, hunger, energy, cravings, digestion, mood, fitness performance). Go back to **The Plan** and review how to address these areas, according to your presentation.

Your body type is relatively sensitive to carbohydrate intake. Therefore, I would suggest you follow the plan outlined in **From High Carb to Low Carb** if you need to decrease your carbohydrate intake. I suggest that the endomorph body type, try zero servings of complex carbohydrates rather than the recommended two servings provided in **The Plan: Calculate Your Caloric Needs.** The endomorphs should get all carb content from vegetables and two servings of fruit. Again, ease into this if you are currently taking in a fair amount of carbs.

After you have figured out the safe amount of complex carbohydrate intake for your body, and after a week of trying this amount, your weight isn't budging, try moving all of your carbohydrates (fruit) to one meal (ideally after a workout, in the am or at dinner). Do this for one week. If things are moving in a favorable direction, stay here. If your weight still is not budging, try taking out a serving or two of fat. Try this for one week. If things are moving and shaking, then stay here.
If not, continue to the next option after a week.

You can also try to change up your eating based on your workouts. On cardio days (yoga, walking, dancing, etc.) have only three meals and zero to one serving of complex carbohydrate. On these days have a lower fat intake as well. On days that you have HIIT training or circuit train-ing, have four meals with two servings of complex car-bohydrate (one after your workout, one at dinner). Again, if things are working after a week, stay here. If your workouts are suffering, you are feeling fatigued through-out the day, or your sleep starts to suffer, then you may need to slowly add in a fruit or a carbohydrate serving, up to 30% of your total intake.

Otherwise, play with your snacks. If you are snacking between meals, play with moving back to three meals per day. If you are eating three meals per day, try adding one snack during the day (especially on days you do weight training or intense exercise).

Once the endomorph approaches their goal weight (within 15 pounds or so), then it may be safe attempt to add in a complex carbohydrate 1/2 serving at a time for one week before adding another 1/2 serving. Again follow the week to week plan outlined in **Low Carbohydrate Lifestyle, Already?** to help you add in your carbohydrates without sabotaging your efforts. Keep your snacks that have sugar in them (even approved cheats such as dark chocolate and red wine) to a minimum of 2-3 times per week or none at all if you are trying to lose more weight. The cleaner your diet, the better.

Applying the Macronutrient Percentages to Create a Menu Plan

Our overall goal in this section is to determine your *daily percentages* of each macronutrient; the *total calories* from each macronutrient that you will need; the *grams per day* of each macronutrient required and the *grams per meal* of each macronutrient that will be necessary. Does this sound confusing? Don't fret. I'll walk you through the process with some straightforward and not-so-intimidating math. Let's use the endomorph somatotype to illustrate the process of creating your macro nutrient parameters for one day.

First, you will need to determine the weight you wish to lose. In this case, our endomorph wants to lose 20 pounds. Because this is more than 15 pounds, we want to start with a lower carbohydrate range. Thus, we will start with 10% carbs.

Next, determine the percentage of fat you want to take in each day. There is a suggested range for you to use as a starting point. In the case for our endomorph, it is 60-70%. Keep in mind that we will need to provide a little wiggle room so that our endomorph can tweak the percentages (within reason). As our endomorph gets a feel for what his or her metabolism responds well to, then it may be necessary to increase calories from fat from 60% to 70 or 80%. Another option is to increase protein to one gram per pound of body weight.

After you determine your carbohydrate and fat intake, the rest of your calories should come from protein. For our endomorph who wants to lose 20 pounds, the rest of the caloric intake will come from protein and will be around 30% of the total calories eaten that day.

Now that you have your carbs percentages of 10% carbohydrates, 60% fat and 30% protein, you will need to determine how to create your meal plan based on your caloric needs.

Let's say that I have determined from **The Plan: Calculate Your Caloric Needs**, that our endomorph will need 1500 calories per day to lose weight. Now that we have this information, we will need to determine how many grams of carbohydrates, fat, and protein the endomorph model will need each day.

> TIP:
>
> *If you want to have a phone app or a website do this for you, there are many from which to choose. I use My Fitness Pal or Cronometer. If you use MFP application, go to your "Goals" page and adjust your calorie and macronutrient goals by customizing the default. Put in the percentages you wish to use and you will get the total grams of each macronutrient you will need to shoot for each day. Or, you can calculate the grams of each macronutrient you will need, with simple math. See the **Macronutrient Calculation Worksheets** in the menu labeled "Resources" at journeytowardjoy.com.*

Calculate Carbohydrate Grams:

0.1 (10%) X 1500 (total calories) = 150 calories from
150 calories \ 4 (calories per gram of carb) = 38 grams of carbohydrates per day.

> **NOTE:** you will need to include fiber in your daily intake. You are looking for NET carbs. Therefore, if

you ate 63 grams of carbohydrate in a day and you logged 25 grams of fiber, then your NET carbs will be 38 grams.

Calculate Fat Grams:

0.6 (60%) X 1500 = 900 calories from fat per day

900 calories \ 9 (calories per gram of fat) = 100 grams of fat per day

Calculate Protein Grams:

150 + 900 (carb + fat calories per day) = 1,050 total calories

1500 (daily total) - 1,050 = 450 calories left over for protein

450 calories \ 4 (calories per gram of protein) = 113 grams of protein per day

Now that we have the total grams of each item, we will need to determine how many grams our endomorph will need for each meal. For the endomorph we will want to shoot for 500-750 calories for each meal, depending on whether the endomorph prefers to intermittent fast with one, two or three meals per day. Otherwise, three meals is a good place to start.

Breakfast (500 Calories Total)

500 x 0.1 (10%) = 50 calories of carbohydrates => 50 calories \ 4 grams = 12.5 grams of carbohydrates (NET CARBS)

500 x 0.6 (60%) = 300 calories of fat => 300 calories \ 9 grams = 33 grams of fat

500 x 0.3 (30%) = 150 calories of protein. 150 calories \ 4 = 38 grams of protein.

Lunch and Dinner (Similar to Breakfast)

So now that we have the calories and gram amounts figured out for our endomorph, we will need to create a menu plan, accordingly. Therefore, we will need to add up the fat, carbohydrate and protein grams of *all* of your food. To help you out, 1/2 cup of sweet potato is about 30 grams of carbs. One tsp of oil is about 5 grams of fat. There are 7 grams of protein in one egg and 35 grams of protein in 4 oz of chicken breast. Some foods, like quinoa, are a mixture, so you'll have to make sure you monitor the details of each macronutrient to get an idea of what you need for each meal to meet your daily needs.

If you choose to calculate your daily macronutrients and monitor each meal individually, then I suggest that you save one day during the week to plan your meals and your snacks. Use your phone app to keep track of your macronutrients at each meal and to monitor your daily intake totals. Logging this information requires a lot of hard work and diligence, so once again, if you simply need an idea how to stay on track with your health, stick to the nutrition guide and serving guidelines in **The Plan: Calculate Your Caloric Needs** and don't worry about macronutrient counting.

However, if you choose to calculate your numbers like the mad nutrient scientist that you are, then keep in mind that even with knowing your body type, you may need to adjust your macronutrient requirements based upon *your* body's metabolism and your response to food. For example, if you try low carbohydrate intake at 10% and lose weight for a few months, then hit a plateau (no movement on the scale for three weeks and no changes in your measurements), then try playing with your intake by increasing your protein intake to 35 or 40%. Or, try upping your fat intake to 70 or 80% See if this moves you in the right direction. You can refer to Breaking through the Plateau if you get stuck (pun very much intended).

Every body is unique and has individual requirements. That is why there is *no* prescribed method of weight loss. Health and wellness must be considered a journey and adventure of trial and error, at times, to determine what your body needs. Viewing weight loss as a journey is more realistic than considering your fitness goals, in their entirety, as a destination. I know that this insight is not necessarily helpful for those of you who need a quick fix. Please keep in mind, the whole intention of this book is to help *you* create the *best* path toward your ultimate health and to follow a path that may, at times, require uphill battles and occasional backtracking. My goal is to help you create the *best route for you* and give you the tools to self-analyze and determine whether to take a left or right turn when you come to crossroads. Of course, you may need to backtrack and explore a different direction, altogether.

In the next chapter, we will get into the fun details of creating an individualized workout plan specific to your body type. The focus is on maximizing efficiency and results while minimizing the amount of effort required. Pretty exciting, huh?

Chapter 13

Fine-Tuning Your Fitness Needs by Body Type

A Method for Creating a Fitness Schedule for the Type "A" Folks Who Need Even More Structure

Using the guidelines provided in **The Plan: Creating Your Workout Routine** will be useful for most people who want to create a customizable, yet feasible plan for improving overall fitness goals (i.e., flexibility, strength, stamina, endurance, balance, speed, etc.). However, if you wish to tailor your routine to fit the needs of your particular somatotype, finding the types of movement that will maximize your results, can be very tricky. Given this challenge, if you have a general idea of what category you fit into (ecto/meso/endomorph), then you have a decent place to start. The key is to understand your goals and to understand the physiology behind different types of exercise. In general, you can expect superior fat burning with High-Intensity Interval Training that will boost your fat burning capabilities for 24-28 hours post workout. Also, you will increase your cardiovascular endurance and stamina if these short workouts are done properly, with intensity and focus.

MON	TUE	WED	THU	FRI	SAT	SUN
back and biceps	45 minute walk	shoulders and triceps	30 minutes yoga	legs and glutes	REST	45 minute walk

You can expect an increase in lean muscle tissue with resistance training. You can build muscle one of two ways: higher weight with lower repetitions until you fatigue the muscle group or you can utilize moderate lower to moderate weights with higher repetitions until you fatigue the muscle group. Depending on your body type, you will choose one of these methods. When performing long bouts of cardiovascular exercise, it is important to choose low impact, slow to moderately paced movements performed for 45 minutes or more. For the sake of utilizing glycogen storage properly and avoided injuries from repetitive movements, all body types will benefit from avoiding intense exercise for extended periods of time (think running, jogging, step aerobics, spinning classes, etc.). If you belong to a gym, consider finding a trainer who is familiar with somatotypes and is interesting in applying your somatotype recommendations to a specified schedule. Now, let's take a look at the different body types and the suggested exercises for each.

Ectomorph Fitness:

- Avoid long cardio sessions as this can cause wasting of lean muscle tissue
- Keep your workouts short, intense and sweet
- 5-6x/wk isolate muscle groups with strength training
- Increase calories to a caloric surplus (above maintenance)
- Don't do too much exercise
- 3-4 sets; 6-12 reps of weight training
- Incorporate lots of rest in between sets

- Do hardcore muscle training with heavier weights
- Eat protein pre and post workouts

To apply this to an actual weekly schedule, it may look something like this:

You have the choice to create your tailor-made routine in your home gym or community gym. However, if you prefer to use a DVD program for at home training, then I suggest a Beachbody® program such as Les Mills Pump and use higher weights on your barbells. Also, Body Beast or Chalene Extreme will benefit you and assist with building muscle without making you look bulky. I am not affiliated with Beachbody® and am not a coach, but I have used many of their workouts and find them to be quite beneficial for transforming the body in a relatively short amount of time.

Mesomorph Fitness:

- Do mostly High-Intensity Interval Training (HIIT).
- Train however you want; however, always mix up your workouts
- Use a combination of weight (dumbbells, resistance bands or body weight) with your cardio workouts.
- Count your macros (I use My Fitness Pal or Cronometer) as your body type is highly sensitive to macro intake
- Use moderate to heavy training 4-5x/wk
- When using resistance weight training, I suggest that you do 4-5 sets of 8-12 reps

- Your rest periods for your HIIT training should be short 15-30 seconds)
- Partake in gentle and long sessions of cardiovascular exercise such as yoga, pilates, and walking; but, you will not need a lot
- Eating at or around maintenance calories can be beneficial, so try this if you have made all of the necessary nutrition adjustments for your body type and you have reached a plateau (or visit the **Breaking through the Plateau** chapter).

MON	TUE	WED	THU	FRI	SAT	SUN
23-30 minutes HIIT focused on lower body	walk 45 minutes	23-30 minutes of HIIT focused on total body	90 minutes of yoga	20-30 minutes of HIIT focused on upper body	REST	15 minutes of HIIT focused on abdominal work; 30 minutes of yoga

The great thing about the mesomorph body type is that it will respond very well to HIIT training and moderate weight lifting in combination with gentle cardiovascular exercise. If you are working in a gym, you may need to create your customized HIIT exercises (see **The Plan: Creating Your Workout Routine**). You can also find plenty of HIIT training workouts on YouTube (see my suggested channels in the **Resources** section of this book). Otherwise, if you prefer to utilize a DVD program, then I recommend that you give Beachbody® a try. For challenging HIIT training, I recommend Focus T25 with Shaun Thomas. For those who are intimidated by a fast paced routine, this program has a wonderful modifier to help you make it through the intense 25 minutes. Also, if you are in relatively decent shape already but looking to take it to the next level, you can review P90X3 (30-minute workouts). Contrary to belief, I would not suggest this program for beginners. It will require far too much modification. If you decide to give it a whirl, you may wish to invest in a resistance band and a door brace for your band to do modified pull-ups. I found the abdominal workout and the HIIT training for Les Mills Combat to be extraordinarily challenging and beneficial. So, if you are looking to add some variety to your routine, it may be worth the investment and you can mix the programs up and create your customized schedule.

Endomorph Fitness:

- Utilize a cardio and weight training combination (think circuit training)
- Do a few low-intensity cardio sessions each week
- Participate in moderate to heavy weight training, 4-5 times per week, using 4-5 sets of 8-12 reps; the idea is to do more sets and more repetitions
- Keep your rest periods shorter (15-30 seconds).
- When using HIIT training, work your upper body more than your lower body, when possible.
- Make sure you are in a caloric deficit.
- Increase protein and get carbohydrates from veggies and limited fruit.

MON	TUE	WED	THU	FRI	SAT	SUN
cross training with cardio and weights	15 minutes HIIT; 45 minutes walking	cross training with cardio and weights	cross training with cardio and weights	15 minutes HIIT; 45 minutes walking	cross training with cardio and weights	REST

For the endomorph, it is important to find fun cardio-driven cross-training programs that involve weight training. As mentioned, the weights should be heavy enough that by 8-12 repetitions the muscle is fatigued. Rest periods should be short and try for 4-5 sets with each muscle group.

Depending on your preference, you can attend a cross-training-like class at your gym. If you like to workout at home, then I recommend a few programs to try. If you like Barre classes, then I recommend Physique 57 video series. These videos are fun, intense and challenging. The upper body exercise utilizes weights, while the lower body exercises use body weight and a playground ball. Also, Les Mills Pump is a good weight-lifting program that is quite the cardiovascular workout and utilizes moderate heavy weights with high repetitions as well. For HIIT training, you may want to try TurboFire HIIT workouts that are part of the program. Also, the upper body HIIT in Les Mills Combat is helpful for the endomorph as it focuses on the right area. You Are Your Own Gym offers an HIIT training that is a total body workout. The beginner workout is free on YouTube at this time.

Now that you have your individualized fitness routine dialed in, I suggest you create your workout calendar based upon your body type's proposed plan. You can print off blank workout sheets from the Resource menu at journeytowardjoy.com.

In the next chapter, we dive into the world of plateau breaking. You can guarantee that you will need at least one suggestion in this chapter as you venture along your fitness journey. You're welcome.

Chapter 14

Breaking through the Plateau

Suggestions on How to Get You Closer to Your Goal

It is inevitable that at some point in your journey toward your health and fitness goals you will experience a plateau. For this book, the definition of a plateau is a length of time in which your fitness progress is at a standstill. Typically, any time greater than three weeks may qualify as a plateau, although many scale-obsessed folks consider a plateau to be a stagnant number on the scale for more than two days. However, the latter method is not fair (or effective) for determining progress. The scale does not measure your body's ability to adapt and to respond to changes in exercise, food intake, and new habits. It is necessary to look at all contributing factors to your progress (beyond a couple of days) to truly gauge how your body is responding. Given the many factors that contribute to improvement, three weeks is my recommendation.

While some folks may find the plateau nothing but frustrating, I can assure you that a plateau is a remarkable gift. It is the body trying to come up with every way possible to keep you from malnourishment; from falling underweight and from dying. Sounds like a good design, right? After all, you can't just lose a half a pound every week for the rest of your life, can you? You would eventually wither away into nothing! A plateau is the body's innate ability to sense the change and do what is necessary to adapt to the modification. Losing weight isn't the body's preferred method of survival, by any means. On the contrary, putting on storage is what the body prefers to protect itself in times of famine.

But you aren't starving yourself, and you aren't trying to do anything drastic (I sure hope not at this point!). So why won't the scale budge? First of all, you need to monitor the physical gains more than the number on your scale. Have your measurements changed? Has your body fat percentage dropped? Are you getting stronger, more flexible and faster in your workouts? These are all indicators that you are indeed NOT plateauing. One can argue that these indicators are much more important than the number on your scale. The scale won't tell you how much lean muscle mass you have put on. It won't tell you if the muscle that you are building is retaining a bit of water. It won't tell you that you ate something the night before that is causing inflammation in your body. It certainly won't tell you about any hormone fluctuations during your monthly cycle (for you women who know what I am talking about). You have to take into consideration the *big* picture.

Let's say that your weight does plateau for a good three weeks and you are not yet at your goal. Assuming your goal is within a healthy range for your body type, then let's work through the appropriate formula for trouble shooting. First, make sure to work through all of the indicators of hormone imbalance (sleep, hunger, energy, cravings, digestion, mood and exercise performance). If you achieve balance with each indicator, then work through the suggestions for stalled fat loss as discussed in **The Plan: Calculate Your Caloric Needs.** Once you have accomplished this and you are still at a standstill, then you are ready for additional tips to get you on your way to busting through the stagnation. These are options and tools for you to try when you don't see any movement in your performance or your weight loss. Because each body is unique, not every option will work for you. Let's review that one more time: Because each body is unique, not every option will work for you!!! I highly suggest that you exercise patience, here. Take *one* option at a time — and at minimum — of one to two weeks, track your progress. If you combine too many options, you won't know what is working for your body. You can track your progress by using the **Progress Trackers** located on the menu item labeled Resources at journeytowardjoy.com.

When addressing a plateau, it is necessary to ALWAYS START WITH FOOD. Weight loss is mostly attributed to diet and macronutrient intake more than fitness. So let's start with making adjustments where it counts.

Reassess Your Caloric Intake!

Take a look at your diet. Chances are your stagnation is due to something going on in the food and drink department. You are going to have to be brutally honest, here. There is no room for "but" and "can't"! There is no room for excuses. First, you need to take a look at your caloric intake. *Have you been charting your daily servings using the* **Meal and Serving Tracker**? *Do you know how many calories you are consuming?* If not, I suggest you use My Fitness Pal for three days and track everything you are eating. *Are you above your caloric goal?* Overconsumption is probably the reason you are not losing weight. If this is the case, get back on track by following your serving suggestions from **The Plan: Calculate Your Caloric Needs.** Do this for two weeks and check for any changes in your measurements or movement on the scale. If either measurements or weight decrease, you have found your new weight loss plateau breaker.

If on the contrary, your calories are below the suggested amount, this too, will assuredly explain your difficulty in losing weight. If your caloric intake dips too low, for too long, your metabolism will very intelligently adjust to the new low to prevent you from wasting away. Your body will very smartly hold on to every morsel of food and fat to eschew starvation. I see this all of the time: women who have been chronic dieters on low-calorie diets, exercising and unable to lose weight. In fact, they usually gain weight using this method. The solution? STOP DIETING! Give your body the fuel it needs, and it will burn the fat you want.

As an illustration, if you put a few sticks in your fire place and lit a match, you may get a flame, but your fire will quickly burn out, and you will not heat up your home. If you slowly add large enough pieces of chopped wood and continually add to the fire when the flames start to die down, you will not only have a blazing fire, but you will heat your entire home, efficiently. Your body is no different. You must give it the fuel it needs (within reason) to create a fat burning furnace; to create a hormone shift that ignites the fat burning capability of the mitochondria in your cells.

What do you do if you have been eating too low of calories you suspect this is the cause? You'll need to rehabilitate your hormones and slowly start to fill your fireplace up with wood and flames. You can't throw a ton of logs in and expect the fire to get big. You've got to coddle it a bit at first and slowly add in one log at a time until it can burn on its own at full capacity. So, slowly add in 100 calories to your current intake, for one week. The next week add in another 100 calories, the next week, etc. Each week, add in this small amount until you reach your maintenance calories. To figure this out, please reread **The Plan: Calculate Your Caloric Needs.**

Once you hit maintenance, you are going to stay there for *at least* two weeks. You may need to stay here a month or two to unequivocally help your body to reignite the hormones that are out of balance—and thus, preventing you from reaching your goal. If you are in a hurry, you may miss the opportunity to help your body nourish itself and rehab the damage done by over-dieting. DO NOT SKIP AHEAD OR PASS GO IF THIS IS YOU! I'm serious! Chronic dieting can stress hormone balance and keep you from reaching your goal. It took an accumulation of time to generate the damage; it will take an assemblage of time to heal. BE PATIENT! Stop trying to get in a hurry to reach your goals. You will get there. It is about the journey, remember? Enjoy the process of healing and nurturing that you are creating. Take pride in the fact that you are making it a priority to care for yourself by giving your body what it needs to thrive.

For those folks who have healthier metabolisms and a nominal history of dieting or damage, you will find that you may lose more weight when you increase calorie intake to maintenance for either two weeks before dropping back down to a healthy deficit. Conversely, you can try eating at maintenance for two to three days per week, alternating with a caloric deficit of 200-300 calories on the other days. This method keeps the body guessing and can often be enough to instigate change.

Reassess Your Food Choices!

You've taken a look at your caloric intake, and you've made sure you are in your Goldilocks spot for caloric intake. If you are on par with this, you will need to dive deeper into your food choices. Be honest with your consumption. *Are you drinking alcohol regularly?* Recall that alcohol can slow down fat loss for 24-48 hours after imbibing. If you have been indulging a bit each week, dial it down to once per week (or none at all), if this is the case.

Have you incorporated complex carbohydrates into your diet? If so, try taking them out (other than fruit and vegetables) for a couple of weeks and see if this helps you. If you have already taken them out, try adding the approved complex carbohydrates back into your diet. Add one serving for a week. If your weight starts to shift in a favorable direction, you may deduce that this is beneficial for you. If the scale numbers remain resolute, try adding in a second serving of carbohydrate, for one week. For some people, it is helpful to keep a low to moderate carb diet with this plan, versus a more ketotic diet (using fatty acids as fuel versus glucose). However, if you choose to add carbohydrates in, make sure you do so slowly and see how you feel. Don't just jump in with both servings of complex carbohydrates (see options provided in **The Plan: Calculate Your Caloric Needs** and **Low Carbohydrate Lifestyle, Already?**). If you have been following the plan without complex carbohydrates, then you will need to make sure that you are paying attention to your body's response to their reintroduction. *Are you feeling hungrier between meals? Are you experiencing more cravings? Is your energy going down after you eat them? Is your mental clarity affected? Did your digestion change for the worse? Has your sleep suffered? Has your workout performance worsened?* Any of these reactions and responses are signs that adding carbohydrates back in may not be the best choice for you at this time. It doesn't mean that you can't enjoy these foods, it just means we are going to have to explore other reasons for your plateau.

Are you tracking your sugar and carbohydrate intake? If you are doing the daily cheats that are allowed, try taking them out for a week. *Are you snacking on any foods that are not on the approved food list? Do you know how many carbohydrates and sugars you are getting each day?* If not, go back to My Fitness Pal or Cronometer and track your food for three days. If you find that your sugar intake is over 30 grams, eliminate the excess. If you find that your net carbohydrate intake (subtract fiber grams from the total carbohydrate grams) is over 75, then you will need to take a look at your sources of carbohydrates each day. Get all of your carbohydrates from green leafy and cruciferous vegetables as well as the approved fruits for a while and see if this changes anything for you. Again, try this for one week and reassess your progress.

Are you eating dairy and nuts? If you have not tested for food sensitivities, I highly suggest that you find a practitioner who will help you identify any food sensitivities you may have. It may be, if you are eating dairy or nuts on a regular basis, this could be causing inflammation in your body—and thus, causing water retention. If you suspect that this could be the culprit, try cutting either dairy or nuts out of your diet, one at a time, for one week and see how you feel and if the scale budges. If so, you know that you are most likely sensitive to these foods, right now.

Reassess the Timing of Your Meals!

If you have gone through the sections above and you have either tried these options or are currently on point with your diet and exercise, then consider changing up your eating window and adopt intermittent fasting. Keep in mind; you will not be changing your caloric intake (although you may find it difficult to get all of your calories packed into a smaller amount of time or fewer meals); but rather, you are changing the timing of your eating. For example, rather than eat a breakfast lunch and dinner, try having a late lunch and an earlier dinner in a six-hour window. So, for instance, you may choose to break your caloric goal into two meals at 12 pm and 6 pm. You can vary the number of hours that you fast, and as a result, you will modify the hours of your eating window. Some days you can try an eight-hour window, other days a four-hour window. See how you feel.

TIP:

It is best to pair intermittent fasting with a history of eating minute amounts of sugar, lower carbohydrate grams, and higher fat grams. For those of you who know you are in ketosis and have confirmed this regularly with a glucometer (I recommend Precision Extra) to measure ketones in your blood, then intermittent fasting will feel very natural to you as you are accustomed to burning your fat for fuel. You want your ketone levels to be between 0.5 and 5; but, 1.5 seems to be ideal according to some experts.

You can also try a 24 hour fast once a week. I like having a big dinner and waiting until the following evening to have another big meal. I drink a little coffee in the am and have tea and water throughout the day. I enjoy the cleansing and detoxifying effect this seems to have. It also helps to rid the body of inflammation that accumulates from time to time. Either way, you can experiment with this method and see how you feel and how your body responds. I must warn you that *not every body will respond favorably (and with fat loss) to intermittent fasting.* Sometimes this type of stressor can increase cortisol and thus create havoc with one's attempt to drop body fat.

> **TIP:**
> *You can assess your body's stress response rather simply with either tracking pupillary response or heart rate variability. With these two methods, you will have a decent idea (without expensive testing) to determine if your body's response to intermittent fasting (or any change you wish to try for that matter) is causing cortisol levels to rise.*

PUPILLARY RESPONSE

To track your pupillary response, take your phone into a room without windows and stand next to the mirror with the lights off. Turn the flashlight on either from your phone or an actual flashlight. Shine the light into one eye, from the side. Your pupil should constrict and remain constricted over 30 seconds. If they dilate again before this time, you may have adrenal stress. Granted this method is not super scientific; but, it can give you a baseline for determining your body's response to a change in your methods (such as starting a fast).

HEART RATE VARIABILITY

Tracking heart rate variability is a rather cool tool for assessing both sympathetic and parasympathetic balance in the body. I recommend that EVERYONE does this. It is possible to train your body to respond more favorably to stressors once you are aware of how your body is reacting (positively or negatively). You can also use heart rate variability to determine if your new method of intermittent fasting is an unfavorable choice for your nervous system at this time. How amazing is that? You get a direct resource in tailoring your habits to fuel fat loss and manage your stress levels! You can try any of the following phone applications: Inner Balance (from HeartMath), bioForce HRV iThlete or HRV4Training app. Keep in mind that some applications require a separate device to help you accurately assess your nervous system's response to stress; but, most will not break the bank. Heck, even some wrist watch fitness trackers have this capability.

Reassess Your Macronutrients!

If you have evaluated your nutrition and your workouts and you don't see results, then you may benefit from taking the somatotype quiz and seeing if your macronutrients need to be adjusted. Some athletic types (mesomorph) may thrive with an increase in protein and a decrease in fat. Also, mesomorphs tend to respond well to increasing their HIIT training, within reason. Thinner types (ectomorph) may find that a slight increase in carbohydrates (again, within reason) and lightening up on their cardio and increasing weight training, help them significantly. The endomorph may benefit from lower carbohydrate intake and increase weight training and long walks or yoga sessions sprinkled in with circuit training. Feel free to review the chapters **Calculation Your Macronutrient Intake For Your Body Type** and **Fine-tuning Your Fitness Needs by Body Type** for details, if you suspect you need to make adjustments for this reason.

Reassess Your Fluid Intake!

If you are not consuming a minimum of half of your body weight in ounces of water per day, then you are going to find losing weight to be challenging from time to time. You cannot expect your body to rid itself of excess toxins, waste materials, and flush fat if you are not providing the cleansing action that makes it all possible. Ideally, you are drinking your full body weight in ounces per day!

Reassess Your Sleep!

We know that most of your body fat burning takes place while you are asleep. If you are having difficulty falling asleep; you wake up often; you go to bed after 10; you wake up feeling groggy, then you most likely are not burning as much fat as possible. Make every effort to correct this problem—not just for your fat loss—but your overall health. See the **Preparing For Success** chapter to get some ideas on how you can improve your sleep without supplements or pharmaceuticals. If these suggestions don't help, then ask your practitioner for a natural recommendation—or better yet, ask your practitioner to determine if you are a candidate for a sleep study. Ruling out sleep apnea is always a necessary method for aiding in long-term fat loss and reducing cardiovascular risk or premature death. Additionally, you may consider testing your overnight cortisol levels to examine your sleep cycle and circadian rhythms. By doing so, you may identify if spikes in cortisol during the night are affecting your sleep. Sometimes, nourishing your adrenals with a few supplements and decreasing stress (in combination with a nightly restorative routine) is enough to set your biorhythmic patterns back on track. The combination of supplements and stress reduction provides a good place to start if testing is not in your budget.

Reassess Your Stress Levels!

Oh, stress! Everyone has some of it, and most people have a lot of it. It is very common to see people with weight concerns that have had stressful events occur in their life. The stress tends to put the body in a "fight and flight" mode—or if the stress is chronic, the adrenals can become so taxed that they no longer produce adequate levels of stress chemicals. The lack of response can occur as a result of being "on high alert" for too long, and the response is weak or lacking. Whether the adrenals are on high alert or barely responding, stress is usually the culprit. Stressors come in many different packages and may be the bi-product of a variety of forms and combinations of triggers. Stressful jobs or the loss of a job, stressful relationships, too much coffee, too much high-intensity exercise, change in income or control of finances, surgery, any infection, any illness (acute or chronic), chronic dieting, chronic cardio, lack of sleep, etc. are all possible stress inducers. There are *many* contributing factors to a person's stress level. If you suspect that stress has been an issue, then it is time to take action. Here are some things I suggest to help you move toward recovery:

Adopt a morning ritual.

To make it easy, I have provided you with my ideal morning ritual at journeytowardjoy.com (Why You Need a Morning Ritual STAT). You can see what I do every morning to ensure that I have a peaceful and productive morning. If you are considering adopting a morning routine, it is necessary to carve out time each morning that is yours and yours alone. During this time (and you choose the length of time from 15 minutes to 2 hours, if you wish) you will need to — at minimum — accomplish rehydration, light stretching or moving, either a short meditation or deep breathing and scheduling your day (if you don't do this at night). If you have time, add journaling in a gratitude journal, reading an inspiring book, prayer, and exercise. Regardless of your timeline or your method, having time set aside that is just carved out for you, every day, will make a significant impact on your outlook for the rest of the day. Don't forget to create an evening ritual as well (see the chapter **Preparing For Success**).

Meditate each day.

Even if you close your eyes and focus on deep breathing for 5 minutes, make it happen. You can use a guided meditation with YouTube or your favorite phone app if you prefer. Being present in the moment is the greatest gift we have. Drink it up and learn from it. The best way to increase awareness of the present moment is to practice mindfulness, and it starts with meditation. Start with 5 minutes each morning. Increase up to 10 minutes, then 10 minutes twice a day, then 10 minutes three times a day. Getting your breath back in order and calming your nerves is the best way to nourish your soul and rehabilitate an overly-taxed body.

Practice yoga and stretch regularly.

If you are not practicing yoga right now, ask yourself why and make it happen. There are so many methods and so many teachers out there that you can find the exact type and personality that suits your needs. Don't like all the spiritual stuff? There's someone out there that will resonate with you. Don't like it because it is too slow? There are faster-paced yoga styles out there. Don't feel you are flexible enough? First of all, that is why you *should* be doing yoga and secondly, find a teacher that provides a lot of modifications that work for you. You should be stretching your body for 15-20 minutes, minimum every day. The quintessential time is before you go to bed and when you get up in the morning.

Use an app to monitor stress.

I like Heart Math Inner Balance to measure heart rate variability to indicate how emotional states are directly affecting your nervous system. Predominately, you are tracking your parasympathetic and sympathetic responses to stress which in simpler terms means that you are connecting the heart and the brain to better assess—and thus, control—your reactions to stress.

Take 24 hours before you decide to address anyone you are frustrated with or who made you angry.

Taking this time will give you perspective and allow you to take a more objective (and much less reactive) approach toward handling the situation. Ask yourself why you are angry. Do you feel others take advantage of you? Disrespected? Helpless? Unloved? Whatever the emotion may be, take the time to feel it. Then take the time to ask yourself if you have control. If the situation is something that is out of your hands, then getting angry does not serve you. Let it go. In turn, do something that that will help you feel in control. Call a friend. Go for a walk. Do a meditation. Listen to jazz. Have some valerian tea. Do a favor for someone or do something altruistic for someone in need. I guarantee you will feel better and calmer. When the 24 hours have passed you will have some new perspective, new wisdom and new insight as to how to best address your concerns if they are still weighing on you. Sometimes, the 24 hours is enough to be able to let it go, completely. But if someone has offended you and it is still ruffling your feathers, address the situation calmly, courageously, respectfully and humbly. Equally important, have the outcomes you want, in mind (and expect these results), before you speak.

Stop getting involved in gossipy conversations or emotionally-charged discussions.

Don't waste your time ranting and raving your opinions at the water cooler or on your Facebook page. Gossip is the quickest way to increase your stress levels. If you find that you just can't help yourself, then seize this opportunity to recalibrate your influence on others and take a break from the group of friends or co-workers that ignite your agitation and melodrama. Furthermore, take a technology fast from the social media or TV shows that get you riled up.

Get counsel.

If you are in a relationship that is causing you stress, then seek help. Everyone can benefit from a qualified, third party individual who can accurately assess your needs and provide insight and feedback into your behavior. If it is your spouse or significant other that causes you stress, then seek help together. If they won't go, then at the very least, treat yourself to a listening ear and get the support you need.

Prioritize your time.

Turn off your distractions. Why do we feel that we need to know when we get a text, e-mail, a phone call, a Facebook friend request, etc.? We wonder why we can't seem to get anything done, yet we feel that we must always be available for everyone else's agenda! Pick two times during the day that you will respond to these messages and stick to a schedule. If it is an emergency, people will know how to track you down. Otherwise, your business and your to-do list are the priority. Once you have tackled them, then you can have the rest of the time to feed the frenzy, if you wish.

Don't start any extremes in your diet or your exercise.

Believe it or not, if you're currently under stress and any of your indicators of hormone imbalance have been affected (sleep, hunger, energy, mood, digestion, cravings or workout performance, etc.), then you can bet that your adrenals are over-taxed. If this is the case, then exercising too hard or going too extreme in your low carbohydrate lifestyle will only prevent weight loss —and in some cases, will cause weight gain, despite your "perfect diet and exercise routine." If you suspect that your body has been under stress or you cannot figure out why you aren't losing weight (or why you are gaining weight), then you will most likely benefit from a laboratory test to determine your cortisol rhythm through the day and evening. With your practitioner's help, you can create a treatment plan that includes healthy stress management, sleep hygiene, eating schedules along with the appropriate nutraceutical or pharmaceutical support to rehabilitate your system. With this information, you can make proactive and strategic changes that will assist you in your short and long term health goals.

If you suspect you have cortisol dysregulation or you have confirmed your suspicions with laboratory testing, then too extreme of a change in your fitness routine or your dietary habits will impede your efforts. You should aim for no more than 2-3 high-intensity interval training sessions per week, keeping them under 30 minutes. The less time is better, here. Consider keeping two servings of fruit and two servings of complex carbohydrates in your diet, aiming for about 75 to 100 grams of carbohydrates per day or 20-30% of your total calories per day. Eating the right kind of carbs is of particular importance if you have tried very low carbohydrate intake and your weight has gone up, or your workouts are suffering because you are tired or you experience muscle fatigue quicker than before. Again, I cannot stress enough (no pun intended) that diet and lifestyle habits must be tailor-made for your body. Not everyone will thrive on insufficient carbohydrate intake. Not everyone will improve their fitness with hard-core and intense 60-minute workouts each day (this isn't a very good idea for most body types). You have to pay attention to your hormone balance by monitoring your sleep, hunger, energy, mood, digestion, cravings, and workout performance. If your measurements are changing for the better and these indicators are in balance, then you are on the right track.

While I believe a low carbohydrate diet can be tailored to benefit almost everyone, there is a myriad of varying methods to consider for each person's body and individual goals. It is always a good idea to start with the recommendations in **From High Carb to Low Carb** if you are transitioning into a lower carbohydrate diet. Once you complete this phase, then move on to **The Plan: Calculate Your Caloric Needs.** Do this plan for at least two months, making sure to track your daily progress in the **Daily Progress Tracker** provided for you in the Resource tab at journeytoward-joy.com. Make sure you give yourself time to become fully adapted to the diet as the first 2-3 weeks for most people can be challenging.

If you are eating lower carb already or you have done **The Plan: Calculate Your Caloric Needs**, and your workouts are suffering, or your weight is not changing (or going up), then you will need to do some serious investigation. It may be necessary to add in carbohydrates to your tolerance level slowly. The best method is to follow the suggestions provided in **The Plan: Calculate Your Caloric Needs** for a prescribed method when you aren't experiencing fat loss. Of course, you must pay close attention to any indicators that your hormones are imbalanced (sleep, hunger, energy, mood, cravings, digestion, and performance) and make the appropriate adjustments. Be sure to log your progress each day in the **Daily Progress Tracker** or the **Food and Reaction Tracker** found in the Resource menu of <u>journeytowardjoy.com</u>. Eventually, you will find the sweet spot wherein your energy and mood remain elevated throughout the day, your sleep is optimal, hunger and cravings are under control, your digestion is on track, and workout performance and measurements are improving.

Regardless, of your method of adjustments, you will become empowered to manage your overall health within the parameters of lower carbohydrate intake. Full ketosis isn't beneficial for every individual (albeit very beneficial for many). Keep in mind, if this is your goal, your body may need some time (for some six months to a year) to adapt fully, rehabilitate stressed adrenals and to allow for weight loss to begin. It depends on the individual (are you tired of me saying this, yet?). When it comes to your health, you can't always be in a hurry if there is much rehabilitation to be done.

Reassess Your Exercise!

To look and feel great, we sometimes go for the most strenuous and challenging workouts we can find. While it is important to challenge your body on a regular basis, if you are frequently exercising with high-intensity, this can cause undue stress and subsequent hormone dysregulation. If you are doing cross fit every day, HIIT training every day, running for extended periods of time, etc. then this may be the reason your body is pushing back and resisting change. If you suspect this is the case, then dial it down. Walk, dance or do yoga in the mornings in a fasted state. Take a longer hike on the weekend or participate in a longer yoga class (90 minutes) or so. Do your HIIT training one to three times during the week, spaced out with enough rest in between these intense sessions. If you are not lifting weights already, start lifting or do a form of body-resistance training for 30-45 minutes two times a week. This schedule will not over-tax you and will provide the benefits you need to change your physique. You'd be surprised how profoundly you can turn the dial for fat loss in the right direction by simplifying your routine and taking it easy most days.

If you suspect that your intense workouts may be contributing to your weight loss stagnation or your increase in body fat, then assess your stress levels with the pupillary response method or with the heart rate variability method. I must warn you that not every body will respond favorably (and with fat loss) to lots of intense exercises. Like intermittent fasting, this type of stressor can increase cortisol and thus create havoc with one's attempt to drop body fat. If you determine that you need to assess your body's stress response to your workouts, you can try tracking pupillary response or heart rate variability as described in more detail under the **Reassess the Timing of Your Meals** section aforementioned above.

Conversely, if your workout routine has not been challenging enough, this too, will contribute to stagnation in your progress. Every three to four weeks, you should be changing your routine to keep your body guessing. If you are not currently practicing any intense exercise (for short durations of time), then I suggest you find a type of HIIT training, Tabata sprints, and circuit weight training to elevate your fitness level. Make sure you establish the exercise method that you enjoy and that works for your body (i.e., doesn't cause stress, strain or injury).

In the next chapter, I will share with you some easy and inexpensive ways that you can add to your health routine. I'm sure that you are aware of the importance of regularly detoxifying your body. But, how often do we take the time to participate in regular cleansing? While doing a quarterly liver detoxification cleanse is highly recommended, given our constant exposure to toxins, I want to provide you with practical ways you can help your liver out on a *daily* basis. Feel free to adopt one (or all) of the suggestions that interest you.

Chapter 15

Daily Detoxification

Simple and Inexpensive Ways to Cleanse Your Body

We all have heard of extensive detoxification programs that involve elaborate powders, drinks, supplements, and routines. And while many of these processes are beneficial to the body, they can be expensive, time-consuming and compliance is often difficult.

To be perfectly honest, I recommend that you participate in a "formal" detoxification process on a regular basis, several times a year. Our world is full of toxicity—in the air we breathe, the water we drink, the cleaning supplies we use, the perfume and lotions we put on our body, the foods we eat contaminated with hormones, pesticides, antibiotics, etc. We are *all* dealing with some degree of toxicity, at any given moment.

But what does detoxification have to do with losing weight? Toxins affect the body's ability to balance blood sugar and metabolize fat. Over time, this may lead to insulin resistance. The accumulation of damage parallels trash collectors going on strike and not picking up the garbage. Waste accumulates, making your house and living environment an unfavorable place to visit.

But how do we realistically detox ourselves on a daily basis? And, how do we do this without breaking the bank? The good news is that it is relatively easy if you are willing to set aside a few extra minutes in your daily routine.

Clean up Your Food Choices

Choosing to eat clean, unprocessed, organic food is a no-brainer when it comes to helping your body work more efficiently; supporting the proper utilization of nutrients and the process of detoxification and elimination. If you choose to commit to a whole foods-centered diet, then make sure that everything you eat comes with a limited ingredient list and that each ingredient can be plucked from the earth or provided by an animal—and theoretically, could be eaten without the assistance of humans in a factory. Chances are if your food choice contains more than a few ingredients and you can't make it at home, it probably is processed. Examples of such foods include dairy products, processed meats, dressings, and condiments. If you are serious about simplifying your diet, try making your dressings and sauces for a few weeks and see how you feel. If you lack the time or diligence to do so, then make smart purchasing decisions when shopping at the local grocery store.

Avoid Alcohol, Sugar, and Caffeine for 30 Days

I know that I have instantly made a few enemies with this statement; but, if you believe that everything in your body is somehow connected, then you'll understand that for proper detoxification to occur, your liver will need a break from common toxins that we often ingest, if not daily. Ideally, for two weeks to a month, give your body a break from these substances.

If you are a caffeine addict, then slowly adjust the morning cup of joe, by using 1/4 to 1/2 decaffeinated coffee. Slowly titrate down every three to four days until you are satisfied with a full cup of decaffeinated coffee. In this manner, you won't lose your morning ritual and your liver (and cortisol levels) will thank you.

If you know you are a sugar addict, then you will need to find alternative sources that give you some satisfaction as you work toward a sugarless lifestyle. Stevia and xylitol are great substitutes if you need something sweet to add to your food and drink choices. Look for your favorite whole food sources that offer desserts made with these sweaters—or even better, make your own.

If you don't think you can give up your nightly glass of wine for 30 days, then you *definitely* should consider doing so. You don't need to be addicted to alcohol, to have a sundered relationship with it. Giving your liver (and your body) a break from imbibing may be just what you need to improve sleep patterns, to wake feeling more rested and to establish more healthy boundaries with your liquid of choice after you have cleansed. If you need something in your hand at an up-and-coming party, consider seltzer water fla-

vored with your favorite flavored stevia drops (I like SweetLeaf®
Water Drops) and a sprig of mint, served in a cocktail glass.

Drink a Liter of Water First Thing in the Morning

Water therapy has been an Ayurvedic practice for many years. In
Sanskrit, the name for morning water therapy is *Usha Paana Chik-
itsa*, which roughly translates to "early morning water treatment."

Dehydration can be directly related to many disease processes or
linked as a secondary symptom. Some conditions such as poor digestion, constipation, migraine headaches, obesity, kidney stones,
hypertension, insulin resistance (and much more) may be alleviat-
ed or diminished, with the simple practice of water therapy in the
morning. How does one practice the healing art of water therapy?

1. Avoid alcoholic beverages the evening before you
   water therapy. Upon waking in the morning, within
   a 20 minute period, drink 1.0-1.5 liters of water
   (equivalent to 4-6 cups). At first, you may need to
   start with 2 cups, take a one minute break, then
   drink two more cups and take another break, then
   finish with 2 cups. Your body will get accustomed
   to the practice over time. If you cannot do the full 6
   cups at first, start with 2 cups and work your way up
   by adding one cup to your routine every two or
   three days.

2. Give your stomach a rest from any food or beverage for 1 hour.

This daily practice over time can help you achieve an improved appearance of your skin, boost your immune system, flush your lymphatic system, assist in your fat loss journey and prevent constipation. By getting your bowels moving you further improve your body's waste management mechanisms.

Drink Hot Water With Freshly Squeezed Lemon

Drinking hot lemon water boosts the kidney's ability to filter toxins and naturally acts as a diuretic. Lemon water is a well-known bile thinner, and bile helps to break down fats. Bile cannot do its job, however, if it is thick and sludgy. Lemon water revitalizes and regenerates the liver, promotes healthy movement of the bowels and keeps waste moving in the proper direction: out of your body. The acids found in lemons (and apple cider vinegar) can help to lower blood sugars and slow down stomach emptying, allowing your body to break down carbohydrates and release insulin appropriately. I like to enjoy a cup one hour after my morning water therapy and as part of a morning ritual.

Drink One Liter (or Two) of Cranberry Water Per Day

Some folks theorize that when the lymphatic system becomes more sluggish, it fails to carry away your body's waste—and as a result, the sludge accumulates in our fat cells. The combination of weak connective tissue that lies on top of fat tissue and the accumulation of waste from a sluggish immune system is the perfect combination for creating the fun lumpy bumpy appearance we all know as cellulite.

Unsweetened cranberry juice has amazing detoxification properties. Cranberry contains active ingredients to aid the elimination of excess water, thus making it a potent diuretic. Flavonoids help to strengthen connective tissue, improving the integrity of the lymphatic system—and as a bonus—dramatically diminishing the appearance of cellulite! Cheers to that!

Try adding 4 oz of unsweetened cranberry juice to 28 oz of water in a 32 0z bottle. Drink this throughout the day, *in addition to* two (2) liters of plain water. Because the cranberry acts as a diuretic, it is important also to drink pure water, separate from your cranberry water, to help flush out toxins and keep you hydrated. Feel free to try the **Cranberry Cleanse Water** in the **Recipes** section of this book.

Bounce on a Trampoline, do Heal Drops or Jump Rope

Ever since the NASA endorsement of mini-trampolining as the best exercise for rehabilitating astronauts after a mission, rebounding has continued to provide well-researched benefits that are nothing short of astounding. Bouncing strengthens the lymphatic system and helps the body rid itself of cellulite. The lymphatic system is your body's fat-processing plant. The lymphatic system is secondary to your circulatory system and transports waste products from your tissues, taking them to the blood stream and eliminating them. Also, your lymphatic tissue manages fluid levels in the body, filters out bacteria and houses white blood cells. It is worthy of noting that the lymphatic system lacks the same pump-like structure that the heart has, to keep it moving. Therefore, the body relies on muscle contraction to move lymph properly. One of the best ways to move lymph is to jump on a mini rebounder for 5-10 minutes per day. Even light bounding with just your heels is enough to adequately move lymph, contract every muscle in your body and to improve the tone and texture of your skin.

How does rebounding work as a cleanser and strengthener of every cell in your body? As one jumps upward, at the top of a bounce, the body is weightless for a moment. All gravitational force and stress on the body is lifted, causing cellular decompression. As the body descends into the trampoline—for a split second—the gravitational pull is multiplied, and each cell is compressed. This repetition—of expansion and compression—forces all cells in your body to adapt to the stress, thus strengthening them, over time. We used to think that gravity was the primary source of aging; however, we now know that astronauts in the absence of gravity, age ten times faster than those folks who remain on earth. Also, folks who regularly partake in gravity-centered exercises are less likely to experience age-related muscular and skeletal degeneration. If you don't have a trampoline, you can practice heal drops by lifting and lowering your heels receptively. You can also use a jumping rope for a similar effect.

Dr. Morton Walker, M.D. explains in his book *Jumping for Health*, the many reasons why you need to add rebounding to your daily routine! Just five minutes a day can provide significant benefit. However, once you start you'll love the way your inner child can't help but smile, and you will want to try 20-30 minutes per day.

According to Dr. Walker, M.D., rebounding has been proven to provide the following health benefits:

▸ Increased respiratory and cardiovascular capacity
▸ Improved circulation—and thus, oxygen to the tissues
▸ Lightening of the workload on the heart by enhancing muscular and valvular fluid exchange.
▸ Reduced levels of arterial blood pressure during exercise
▸ Decreased the higher blood-pressure period after exercise
▸ Increased red-cell production activity of the bone marrow (raising oxygen-delivery capacity)
▸ Strengthening of the heart muscle (and all muscles), causing them to work with greater efficiency
▸ Stimulation of metabolic activity
▸ Promotion of growth and tissue repair
▸ Tonification of the endocrine system, especially the thyroid, to increase output

- Enhancement of the body's alkaline reserve for potential emergency output
- Conservation of physical strength and efficiency
- Improvement in coordination through enhanced transmission of nerve impulses and muscle response
- Increased muscle fiber tone
- Provision of relief from neck and back pains, headaches and pains due to poorly toned physiology
- Enhancement of digestion and elimination
- Stimulation of lymph flow for increased immunity and cold/allergy prevention; enhancement of waste-cleansing as mentioned above (think less cellulite and improved immunity)
- Promotion of more restful sleep and relaxation

If you need just one exercise to stretch and tone muscle and improve cardiovascular health, this is the only equipment you need. For those of you with joint issues or who are overweight and prefer modified exercises, this is a safe alternative for you. Indeed, you should check with your physician if you are unsure whether or not you should try rebounding.

Dry Brush Your Skin Before You Take Your Shower

Dry skin brushing is an inexpensive and practical way to provide whole-body benefits in your healthy daily routine. Your skin is your largest organ and responsible for eliminating waste around the clock. However, if your skin is brimming with dead skin cells and toxins, it cannot effectively do its job. Dry skin brushing helps stimulate your lymphatic system—as aforementioned in this chapter—which acts as the sewer system of your body, carrying waste, toxins, and debris away from your tissues. The waste dumps into your circulatory system for elimination. If your sewer system is backed up, this can lead to congestion, inflammation, and disease. Moreover, without a pump (like your heart) to move the sewage, your lymphatic system needs all of the help it can get.

In addition to eliminating waste materials from your tissues by stimulating your lymphatic system, dry skin brushing aids in exfoliating and clearing clogged pores. The act of exfoliation increases circulation to the skin; thus, reducing the appearance of cellulite by preventing the breakdown of connective tissue. Some folks hypothesize that dry skin brushing may improve digestions and kidney function as well.

How do you dry skin brush? You can purchase an inexpensive "back brush" made with natural bristles. The bristles should be on the stiff side, and the handle should be long enough that you can reach your back dexterously. Dry brushing is exactly that: without any water and performed when both your skin and the brush are dry. Brush in light but firm strokes that leave your skin pink but not irritated. Your strokes should be a wiping motion, in one direction, toward your heart. Brush your entire body starting with the soles of your feet and work your way up to your neck, avoiding your face and genitals. For the abdomen and the breasts, some recommend moving in a clockwise formation. From toes to neck, it should take you no longer than two minutes; but, you can take as long as twenty minutes if you have the time.

Oil Pulling

Oil pulling is yet another ancient Ayurvedic practice that will assist in maintaining strong teeth, create an alkaline environment in the mouth (higher pH)—which in turn—discourages the growth of unwanted bacteria and fungus, heals inflamed or bleeding gums and may even balance the body. Some people have reported that it is an effective treatment for reversing tooth decay, although the research is still unclear. Because of its antibacterial and anti-fungal properties, infection is less likely to occur in your teeth and gums; therefore, preventing secondary infection and inflammation from the waste products created by these nasty little buggers.

Oil pulling is the act of swishing your mouth with oil (I recommend virgin coconut oil) for up to 20 minutes. An excellent way to fit this in your day is to put a teaspoon of oil in your mouth before your morning shower. By the time you finish your shower, put on lotion and deodorant, dress, etc. you will certainly have swished for at least 20 minutes. When swishing, try to relax your jaw so as not to fatigue your muscles too much. At first you may find that your jaw tires a bit; but, over time, you will strengthen these muscles and adapt to longer swishing times. When you finish, spit the residue in the garbage or outside. Spitting the oil down your sink may eventually cause unwanted buildup in your pipes.

What else?

If you are interested in a physician-assisted detoxification program, you can find many practitioners who are ready and willing to assist you. Most holistic practitioners have training in gentle detoxification and can provide the appropriate testing mechanisms if you need to identify oxidative stress or metal toxicity, etc. It is always a potent to plan for a 10-21 day cleanse several times a year as a reboot of your system. A change of the seasons is always a great reminder that it is time to rehabilitate your liver, kidneys and other elimination systems.

Conclusion

When I first started writing this book, the intent was to help my friends and family members understand and apply the principles that I used to lose weight, change my body composition and improve my lifestyle. Nevertheless, the deeper I dove into my research and spoke to dozens of patients about their weight loss frustrations, I realized that there were patterns in need of more exhaustive investigation. Conventional low carbohydrate or high-fat diet plans insufficiently address these trends.

You see, the majority of people I meet who struggle with weight are not folks with unhealthful lifestyles. Most are attempting to cut out fast foods and some sugar, they have a relatively active lifestyle, and they are trying to watch how much they eat. Almost everyone I meet with weight-related concerns has a history of stress—or adaptation imbalance to— stress. Folks either present with clear-cut symptoms or with a subclinical presentation recognizable with proper testing. It is entirely too common that people are unknowingly eating foods from time to time or on a regular basis that mount an immune response, causing micro damage to the intestinal walls—and thus, creating local and systemic inflammation. Far too commonly, most folks feel like their energy is not where they would like it to be part of (or most of) the day. And, it is incredibly common that folks are having trouble sleeping — either falling asleep or staying asleep. Even worse, they aren't feeling rested upon waking. You see, all of the commonalities that I see in "most" people, as described above, are exactly that: *very* common. If bringing these things to light so that you feel you are not alone, is a comfort to you, then I have done my job.

For these reasons, I highly suggest that as you embark on a weight loss journey, you seek help in identifying the cause of the weight loss resistance or the weight gain. Most holistic practitioners that specialize in functional medicine will be happy to help you determine where you need help, first. While it is entirely possible that the practical lifestyle adjustments provided in this book will get most people 80% or more toward better health and hormone balance, it is always beneficial to get targeted support with proper testing and supervision with a practitioner that you trust.

I have provided some of the tests I like to use in my practice for you to review in the **Resources** section of this book; but, please know that there are many out there that are just as effective. Feel free to discuss this list with your practitioner and create a treatment plan based on your individual needs. Keep in mind, that if you don't identify the cause of the weight gain, you are merely putting a band-aid on a knife wound. You may stop the bleeding a bit; but ultimately, your body requires stitches. In other words: you may lose some weight by changing your diet and exercise habits; but, if you do not address the root cause of your weight gain, your weight loss will not be permanent or meet your ideal expectations.

In addition to the many physical barriers that a body may have to weight loss, I find that when I investigate further, I frequently find that there is a mental barrier; a mind-body disconnect with the way the person wants to feel and look. Commonly, individuals seeking weight loss have conditioned their mind with negative self-talk and a negative body image. If I could record my interactions with my dear friends, family members, and patients, you would hear a lot of statements such as:

"I've become so fat. I hate it."
"My body doesn't like me anymore."
"I just want to get rid of my gut."
"Nothing fits me anymore."
"I don't want you to take my picture."
"I don't even know if losing weight is possible."
"I've done everything I can, but nothing works."

Folks, this breaks my heart, every time. I get it. I understand. I've been there. When you don't like what you see, and you feel helpless, it does seem impossible. My dear friends, we must change this! We must rise above—and together, change the way we look at ourselves and our future. We cannot continue to participate in degrading thoughts, beliefs and behaviors that are contrary to our designed purpose; contrary to that which we are capable. I am so incredibly passionate about this that I chose to address the topic within the first few pages of this book. But, if you skimmed through this section or you dismissed it altogether and jumped ahead to The Plan, *you are missing the point*!

This book is *not* a catch all for all body types and metabolisms. It is *not* meant to be a miracle method that provides you with the ability to walk a runway or grace the cover of Sports Illustrated or Men's Health with your presence (although with the right training, diet and set of beliefs, these accomplishments can be possible). The purpose of this book is *not* to provide a brain dump of "what I know" to establish myself as one who has all of the answers (although I continue to inquire and investigate, daily).

The intended goal of providing you with this compact information is to teach you practical ways that you can use, today, to rebalance your mental, hormonal and physical landscapes. You now have the tools necessary to give your mind and body a self-actualized makeover. You can achieve this simply by making better choices each day. Your choices will guide you in creating new thought patterns that impact how you view yourself in this world. You now have the tools necessary to make intelligent food purchases. You know the steps necessary in assessing eating patterns and how to modify these patterns to create the best hormonal outcome. You can eliminate the guesswork when determining how you should train your body. You can apply practical methods when you need to manage your stress. Think of this book as providing the ultimate empowerment to learn new ways to take care of yourself. By providing this information, I am passing you "the baton of information" knowing that this information will help you to feel in control. You now have the knowledge that will guide your efforts in addressing some of your health concerns.

MY FINAL THOUGHTS

We have become a society that is over-stressed and poorly adapted to stress. We have been conditioned to believe that we need carbohydrates to survive. We are addicted to our sugary snacks. We have dieted too much in our past, or we have over-trained our bodies. We aren't sleeping well. We are losing touch with how intertwined our mind, body, and soul are. We have lost sight the intricate design of our bodies. We have mistakenly presumed that weight loss is solely dependent upon caloric intake and activity level. We choose to ignore the science in an effort to find the latest diet trick that claims to rapidly take off the weight.

If you don't believe that all metabolic dysfunctions directly connect with the extreme frustration from the consequential weight gain, then I haven't properly communicated the purpose of this book, whatsoever! In putting this eating, exercising and lifestyle plan together, I have all of these connections in mind. You see, it is possible to bring your body back to balance and to reverse any metabolic damage that has amassed over the years. It is possible to reverse engineer (and prevent) the genetic expression of the diseases and metabolic dysfunctions that family members carry within their DNA. It is possible to reverse engineer your "programmed future" to be absent of these health concerns, should you make the right changes. But, it *will* take some time.

To see a lasting change we need to change our mindset and the way in which we talk to ourselves each day. We have to learn to remove the temptation and roadblocks in our pantry, in our home and in our lives that prevent us from moving closer to our goals. We must make better choices when it comes to food. We must eat more (for most of us) and consume more fat and less sugar. We need to train smarter, not harder. We must find ways to address and improve upon our adaptation to stress. We must establish healthful habits at night that enhance our sleep, not deprive us of this vital fat-burning time. We need to develop daily habits to cleanse, detoxify and nourish our system. We need to seek professional help if we are experiencing resistance after attempting these methods. We need to recognize that some imbalances must be corrected if we are to progress in our efforts.

You, my friend, are smart and you want to recognize the patterns in your life—both beneficial as well as those that do not serve you— and change the patterns that are not leading you toward progress. You want to make changes that will move you further in your journey toward being healthier and happier with your physique —and more importantly, with your well-being and quality of life, as you age. You recognize that stress, eating habits, sleep, outlook, digestion and a history of dieting and weight gain are all connected. Simply stated: you cannot address one area without addressing the others.

So, I commend you for taking the steps necessary to reevaluate what you want for yourself. I congratulate you for taking the time to read the pages of this book. I am truly grateful that you have trusted me this far; that you have (hopefully) applied a few of the science-based observations and concepts.

Remember, your health journey is exactly that: a journey. When you lose sight of what you are accomplishing day to day; how you feel; how you are subtly changing (inside and out), you will miss out on the joy that comes from being in control and from knowing you are doing something beneficial for yourself. If you focus on the outcome you want without appreciating your progress, you will only be disappointed and frustrated that you haven't reached your goal.

So, *slow down*. Be thankful every day for the gift of life; the gift of health; the gift of changing your mind and the gift of having the ability to make small adjustments in your lifestyle. Appreciate these things, every day. Roll around, wrestle, play and submerge yourself in them. The more you revere what is right in front of you as you stand in the mirror, the more you will work with your body, not against it—and as a result, begin to see lasting change. Trust me. I see it all of the time.

Again, thank you for taking time out of your journey to read these pages and to consider the science that can help you forge your next steps. May you continue to find joy in your transformation into a Forever Fat Burner.

With much love and respect to you, my friend,

Dr. Linné

Supercharge your health. Simplify your lifestyle. Satisfy your soul.

PART 4
RECIPES AND RESOURCES

Recipes
My Favorite Go-To's

These are all of my favorite recipes that I have been regularly making over the years. The list gets bigger and bigger as I try new things. I suggest you do the same and start creating a list of new foods you enjoy by exploring new recipes. Feel free to peruse my suggested cookbooks in the **Resources** section of this book for some of my top favorites.

It is important to note that I have included recipes that have fruit and complex carbohydrates. Therefore, make sure that you are following your specific guidelines for these food groups, before you plan your meals. For example, if you are just starting this journey and you have been eating carbohydrates and sugar for some time now, then you will need to follow the plan as outlined in the **From High Carb to Low Carb** chapter of this book. The recipes with quinoa, sweet potato, fruit, plantains, almond flour, etc. will be helpful for your transition into the lower carbohydrate, higher fat lifestyle.

If you are already following a lower carbohydrate diet or are choosing to jump right in, then you will choose the approved complex carbohydrate foods once in a while as outlined in the **Low Carbohydrate Lifestyle, Already?** chapter.

Chocolate Berry Smoothie *

A smoothie is my go-to morning meal on days I am craving fruit. I either have it for my breakfast or after my workout. You'll find that you will look forward to the satisfaction of a little chocolate and a lot of nourishing vitamins and minerals.

1 cup unsweetened almond milk or coconut milk (in a carton, not can).

1 serving chocolate protein powder (I like Orgain® vegan chocolate protein powder or Vega® chocolate protein powder found at Costco.com).

3/4 cup frozen berries (blackberries or raspberries)

2 cups power greens (kale, spinach, chard, etc. I buy the large bags at Costco)

1 TBL hemp seeds

1 TBL chia seeds

*1 scoop Amazing Grass® Green Superfood

*1 scoop probiotic or open a capsule into the blender

*1 TBL raw maca powder

- Put all items in a high powered blender for 20-30 seconds until well blended.
- All elements that are optional (*) are worth giving a try (if you want that extra-healthy-super-power thing)!

MAKES ONE (1) SERVING

Per serving: 1 protein, 1/2 complex carb, 1 fruit, 2 vegetable, 1 nut/ seeds

Kale Smoothie

Are you having difficulty getting in all of your veggies? No problem! This shake is my go-to when I want a powerhouse vegetable kick. You can easily fit in 4-6 servings of vegetables in one sitting!

1 cup unsweetened almond milk or coconut milk (in a carton, not can).

4-6 cups baby kale leaves

3-4 dashes of cinnamon

Six drops of liquid stevia

*1 scoop Amazing Grass® Green Superfood

*1 scoop probiotic or open a capsule into the blender

▸ Put all items in a high powered blender for 20-30 seconds until well blended.

▸ All elements that are optional (*) are worth giving a try (if you want that extra-healthy-super-power thing).

MAKES ONE (1) SERVING

Per serving: 1/2 complex carb, 4-6 vegetable

Raspberry Cream Smoothie

This smoothie often ends up being my afternoon snack or my desert, if I need one!

1 cup unsweetened almond milk or coconut milk (in a carton, not can).
1 cup frozen or fresh raspberries
1/4 cup of Great Lakes Collagen Hydrosylate® protein powder
3-4 dashes of cinnamon or pumpkin pie spice
Six drops of liquid stevia
*1 scoop probiotic or open a capsule into the blender

- Put all items in a high powered blender for 20-30 seconds until well blended.
- All elements that are optional (*) are worth giving a try (if you want that extra-healthy-super-power thing).

MAKES ONE (1) SERVING

Per serving: 1/2 complex carb, 1 protein, 1 fruit

Coconut Creamy Chocolate Coffee

16 oz freshly brewed organic dark roasted coffee
1 TBL virgin coconut oil or NOW® MCT oil
1 TBL Kerrygold® butter
Two dashes sea salt

1/4 Tsp vanilla extract

One scoop Orgain® chocolate protein powder

6-8 drops vanilla cream or chocolate flavored stevia

Two dashes cinnamon

- Put all ingredients into a blender.
- Top the blender with a towel.
- Blend for 20-30 seconds until you have a nice frothy foam at the head of the mixture.
- Pour into your favorite coffee mug and top with cinnamon.
- Serve warm.

MAKES ONE (1) SERVING

Per Serving: 1 protein, 2 oil/butter

Basic Keto Coffee

I have this lovely, creamy drink almost every day. There is something so satisfying and energizing with having healthy fats first thing in the morning.

16 oz freshly brewed organic dark roasted coffee
1 TBL virgin coconut oil or NOW® MCT oil
1 TBL Kerrygold® butter

- Put all ingredients into a blender.
- Top the blender with a towel.

- Blend for 20-30 seconds until you have a nice frothy foam at the head of the mixture.
- Pour into your favorite coffee mug and top with cinnamon.
- Serve warm.

MAKES ONE (1) SERVING

Per Serving: 2 oil/butter

Keto Chai

I love this as a coffee alternative when I prefer not to drink coffee!

16 oz unsweetened almond, hemp or coconut milk
Two tea bags of rooibos chai tea cooked in 1/2 cup boiling water
1/2 Tsp vanilla
1 TBL Kerrygold® butter
1 TBL coconut cream, coconut oil or NOW® MCT oil
One scoop stevia powder or 4 drops of liquid

- Let the tea brew for 5-10 minutes.
- Put all ingredients into a blender.
- Top the blender with a towel.
- Blend for 20-30 seconds until you have a nice frothy foam at the head of the mixture.
- Pour into your favorite coffee mug and top with cinnamon.
- Serve warm.

Per Serving: 2 oil/butter

Egg Muffins

Egg muffins (or cups) are a great grab-n-go breakfast choice for those mornings when you are short on time!

12 large eggs
1 (10 oz bag)spinach, chopped
1/2 cup chopped mushrooms
One medium pepper, chopped
One clove garlic
1/2 medium onion chopped
sea salt, black pepper
* chopped basil or cilantro are optional

- Heat oven to 375 degrees Fahrenheit.
- Coat a 12 cup muffin tray with coconut or olive oil spray.
- Whisk eggs together with salt and pepper.
- Add in vegetables.
- Pour into muffin cups.
- Bake approximately 20 minutes or until an inserted fork comes out clean.

MAKES SIX (6) SERVINGS

Per Serving: 1 protein, 1 vegetable

Quick Quiche

Note: without the cheese, chilis, or veggies, you can use this recipe to make Dutch Babies or German pancakes.

1 cup unsweetened almond or coconut milk (carton, not canned)

One 4 oz can green chilis

1/4 cup SIFTED coconut flour

1/3 cup tapioca flour

8 eggs

1/2 cup grated sheep Manchego or cheese of your choice

2 sliced up organic chicken sausage, sliced horizontally into "coins" and cooked 2-3 minutes on each side

1 cup chopped veggies of your choice (jalapeño peppers, mushrooms, onions, spinach, broccoli, etc.) chopped

2 TBL Kerrygold® grass fed butter, coconut oil or avocado oil

1/2 Tsp sea salt

▸ Heat oven to 375 degrees.

▸ Place a 9-inch iron skillet or oven-safe quiche pan with butter into the oven for 5 minutes or until butter is melting.

▸ Blend milk, flour, eggs, cheese and salt in a blender for 20 seconds or until mixed well.

225

- Stir in veggies and pour into your skillet or pan and cook for 30 minutes or until a fork inserted comes out clean.

MAKES FOUR (4) SERVINGS

Per Serving: 1 protein, 1/2 complex carb, 1/2 healthful fat, 1.5 Tsp oil/butter

Eggs Bacondict

Who doesn't love a great excuse to eat bacon from time to time? Add in some eggs, and a tomato and you have a satisfying breakfast. If you're famished, you can add some almond flour pancakes to the mix.

One beefsteak tomato

4 eggs

4-6 strips of uncured, low-sugar, hormone/antibiotic free, organic bacon (Trader Joe's® has smoked salmon bacon that is divine on top of eggs!)

One large avocado

2 TBL apple cider vinegar or white vinegar

1/2 Tsp sea salt

Three egg yolks

1 TBL freshly squeezed lemon juice

1/2 cup plus 2 TBL Kerrygold® butter

One package of frozen chopped spinach

One sweet onion, chopped

*fresh flat leaf parsley, chopped

*smoked paprika

- Heat oven to 375 degrees.
- Place a sheet of parchment paper on a cookie sheet. Place the bacon on the parchment paper.
- Put the bacon in the oven and cook for 17-18 minutes, until the bacon looks thoroughly browned and crispy, but the edges remain unblackened.
- While the bacon is cooking, but the large beefsteak tomato into four equal parts.
- In a saucepan, bring about 2-3 inches of water to medium heat until bubbles begin to form, but it is *not* fully boiling. Add the vinegar to your hot water.
- Carefully break each egg into a separate cup and slowly pour each egg into your saucepan. When all eggs are in, let them sit for 3 minutes. When the eggs become opaque and feel firm to the touch, they are ready. Using a slotted spoon, gently lay each egg on a paper towel to dry.
- In a blender, put the egg yolks, lemon juice, and salt in a blender on medium speed for 30-45 seconds.
- In a double boiler or a pan over a saucepan of boiling water, melt the 1/2 cup of butter.
- With the blender is running, add the hot butter through the hole in the lid *very* slowly at a steady pace, until the mixture has slightly thickened. You can keep the sauce warm by placing it back into the buttered pan over boiling water and maintain a warm stove top.

- Put the frozen spinach in a strainer and run warm water over the leaves. Once the leaves are no longer frozen, press all of the excess water out of the spinach leaves.
- In a skillet, put the chopped spinach, chopped onion and 2 TBL of butter. Warm the ingredients on medium heat until the onions are fully cooked.
- Once your bacon thoroughly cooks, cut the bacon into 1/4 inch bits with kitchen shears.
- Cut the beefsteak tomato into 1/2 inch thick slices. Top the tomato with 1/4 cup of the spinach mixture. Place each egg on top of the spinach and 1/2 inch tomato slice. Add a couple of tablespoons of hollandaise sauce and top with the bacon bits. For more fun, add fresh slices of avocado and garnish with cilantro or parsley. Sprinkle with smoked paprika.

MAKES TWO (2) SERVINGS

Per Serving: 2 protein, 4 oil/butter, 2 healthful fat, 1/2 vegetable

Almond Flour Pancakes *

I love the occasional breakfast with pancakes, eggs, and bacon. When you need something "carby" without going overboard, these are your best friend. If you prefer savory, then forgo the stevia, cinnamon, and vanilla. Replace these with a tsp of your favorite all-purpose seasoning, 1/4 cup of almond cheese or parmesan (if you can do dairy). Top your savory pancakes with fresh avocado and butter. Who's hungry?

1/2 cup almond flour (not meal)

1/4 Tsp baking powder

1/4 Tsp baking soda

1/8 Tsp sea salt

1/4 Tsp cinnamon

Four scoops of stevia powder (or 1 dropper-full of liquid or 1 packet)

Two large eggs

1/4 cup unsweetened coconut or almond milk

1 Tsp vanilla extract

1 TBL coconut oil

Yacon syrup or Lakanto® maple syrup (found on Amazon).

- Heat a large skillet over medium heat with the coconut oil.
- Mix all dry ingredients.

- Whisk all wet ingredients together in a separate bowl.
- Add the wet ingredients and dry ingredients together.
- Drop 2 TBL or 1/8 cup of batter at a time onto the heated skillet
- When edges the brow, flip the pancake and wait a minute or two.
- Serve warm with Kerrygold® butter, your favorite nut butter, yacon syrup or Lakanto® maple syrup.

MAKES TWO (2) SERVINGS

Per Serving: 1 protein, 1/2 oil, 1 complex carb

Quinoa Cakes *

There is something so comforting about pancakes. Having options that are grain free are entirely necessary when you need a good carb fix. If you want something more savory, forgo the cinnamon, vanilla, stevia, banana, and syrup. Add in diced onion, 1/4 of parmesan cheese and top with a little Kerrygold® butter. But, don't forget, make sure you only use quinoa as recommended by your stage of this program.

*1/2 cup cooked quinoa
Two whole eggs
One dash Himalayan salt
1/4 Tsp cinnamon or pumpkin spice
1/2 Tsp vanilla
One scoop dry stevia powder (or 4 drops of liquid)
1/2 Tsp Bragg's® apple cider vinegar

1 TBL tapioca starch, almond flour or coconut flour

1/4 Tsp baking soda

1tsp *almond butter (optional)

1/2 *mashed ripe banana (optional sweetener and thickener)

One serving *Berry Syrup (see recipe)

▸ Place quinoa eggs, salt, cinnamon, vanilla and stevia in a bowl and whip until all ingredients are mixed.

▸ Spray a medium sized pan with coconut oil spray on medium heat.

▸ Spoon out about a 1/4 cup of batter into the pan.

▸ Cook 1-2 minutes until bubbles form on top.

▸ Flip with a spatula and cook for another 30 seconds or so.

▸ Top with the one tsp of almond butter and berry syrup.

MAKES ONE (1) SERVING OF 5-7 PANCAKES

Per Serving: 1 carbohydrate, 1 protein, 1 fruit (if you added the banana), 1 Tsp oil/butter

Sweet Potato Pancakes *

*1/2 cup roasted sweet potato. I like Murasaki from Trader Joe's®. Make sure you are buying sweet potatoes (golden butter-colored inside), not yams (orange). 45 minutes at 375 degrees should be long enough to roast them. You'll know that they are ready when a fork easily pierces through the potato.

Two whole eggs

One dash Himalayan salt

1/4 Tsp cinnamon or pumpkin spice

1/2 Tsp vanilla

One scoop dry stevia powder (or 4 drops of liquid)

1/2 Tsp Bragg's® apple cider vinegar

1 TBL tapioca starch, almond flour or coconut flour

1/4 Tsp baking soda

1 Tsp *almond butter (optional)

1/2 *mashed ripe banana (optional sweetener and thickener)

One serving *Berry Syrup

- Remove skins from potatoes.
- You may need to mash the potatoes for a bit with a fork to get them smooth.
- Add the eggs, salt, cinnamon, vanilla, and stevia in a bowl and whip until all ingredients are mixed.
- Spray a medium sized pan with coconut oil spray on medium heat.
- Spoon out about a 1/4 cup of batter onto a large skillet.
- Cook 1-2 minutes until bubbles form on top.
- Flip with a spatula and cook for another 30 seconds or so.
- Top with the one tsp of almond butter and Berry Syrup.

MAKES ONE (1) SERVING OF 5-7 PANCAKES

Per Serving: 1 carbohydrate, 1 protein, 1 fruit (if you added the banana), 1 Tsp oil/butter

Berry Syrup *

1/2 cup berries

2 TBL water

1 TBL arrowroot powder

6-8 drops liquid stevia (or 1 TBL xylitol)

▸ Warm the berries with two TBL of water and 6-8 drops of stevia or 1TBL of Xylitol in a small sauce pan over medium heat.

▸ Add the arrowroot powder once the mixture starts to boil.

▸ Once the mixture begins to boil, whisk it thoroughly until smooth.

▸ Remove from heat and top off your pancakes.

MAKES ONE (1) SERVING

Per Serving: 1 fruit

Mini Pizzas Crusts *

This lovely and useful recipe is from my dear friend and nutrition expert, The Healing Cave Lady (www.healingcavelady.com). You can use this recipe to create taco shells, gyro-like sandwich wraps to load with some melt-in-your-mouth beef (see stew recipe) or use it as the crust for your favorite pizza toppings. The options are endless.

One large egg

2 TBL sour cream and add water until you reach the 4 oz or 1/2 cup mark

1/4 cup avocado oil, coconut oil or melted Kerrygold® butter

1 cup tapioca flour (or starch). Do NOT substitute.

1/2 Tsp sea salt

1/2 cup cheese (feel free to mix up the cheese type, like parmesan and sharp cheddar).

- Heat oven to 400 degrees.
- Line a cookie sheet with parchment paper.
- In a blender, blend all ingredients (except cheese) until well mixed.
- Add cheese and pulse a few seconds.
- Pour batter onto cookie sheet in approximately 5-inch pancake circles.
- Cook for about 20 minutes until slightly golden.
- Cover with pizza sauce, more cheese, Applegate turkey pepperoni, and chopped veggies of your choice and put back in the oven until cheese melts.
- Or freeze the mini crusts for sandwich wraps for later.

MAKES APPROXIMATELY FOUR (4) SERVINGS OF 2 MINI PIZZA CRUSTS

Per serving: 1/4 of the batter = 1 seeds/dressing, 1 complex carb, 1/2 healthful fat

Mexican Quinoa Rice *

1 TBL avocado oil

4 cups precooked quinoa (follow directions on bag)

1 Tsp chili powder

1 Tsp cumin

1/2 Tsp smoked paprika

1-2 TBL coconut aminos

1/2 Tsp chipotle powder OR 1 - 12 oz can La Costeña® chipotle pepper in adobo sauce

1/3 cup freshly chopped cilantro

sea salt to taste

- In a large skillet heat oil over medium heat.
- Add quinoa and stir the mixture often until the quinoa is warm.
- Add spices, coconut aminos and cilantro.
- Salt to taste.

MAKES EIGHT (8) SERVINGS

Per serving: 1/2 cup = 1 complex carb

Sweet Potato Sausage Hash *

Four organic chicken sausage (casings removed)

4 TBL coconut oil

Two large Murasaki sweet potatoes

1 cup cubed butter nut squash

One large red onion

One sweet red pepper, chopped

Three sprigs freshly stripped thyme

Three sprigs freshly stripped rosemary

Sea salt and black pepper to taste.

1 Tsp smoked paprika or 1/4 Tsp chipotle powder

1/2 cup chicken stock

- Preheat oven to 375.
- Cut sweet potatoes into 12-inch cubes
- Mix all ingredients in a bowl and transfer to a parchment paper-lined cookie sheet.
- Cook until sausage, potatoes and squash are browned (approximately 25-30 minutes).

MAKES FOUR (4) SERVINGS

Per serving: 1 serving = 1 protein, 1/2 vegetables, 1 oil/butter, 1 complex carb

Easy Chicken Sausage Bowl *

1 and 1/2 cups mixed greens

1/2 sweet red pepper, chopped

1/2 cup quinoa, cooked

1 Adele's® organic chicken sausage

1 Tsp avocado oil

2 TBL homemade dressings of your choice (see recipes)

- Heat a skillet over medium heat with avocado oil.
- Slice the sausage into coin-sized pieces and cook evenly on both sides until golden brown.
- Add the quinoa (feel free to spice the quinoa up with your favorite seasonings, fresh herbs and salt and pepper to taste).
- Once the quinoa is warmed slightly toasted, transfer to a bowl filled with mixed greens.
- Top with 2 TBL of your favorite homemade dressing.

MAKES FOUR (4) SERVINGS

Per serving: 1 protein, 2 vegetables, 1 oil/butter, 1 complex carb

Coconut "Rice"

**One bag frozen or fresh cauliflower rice (from Trader Joe's®)
or put one cauliflower head, chopped, into the food processor
and mix until the size of grains of rice**

1/2 cup coconut milk

2 TBL coconut oil

1 TBL coconut aminos

1/4 cup freshly chopped basil

*1 Tsp chili pepper flakes

One medium onion, finely chopped

One scallion sliced thinly

black pepper, sea salt to taste

- In a large skillet melt the oil and sauté the onion with the chili pepper flakes.
- Add salt and pepper and the cauliflower and coconut milk.
- Cook another 5-10 minutes until the coconut milk is absorbed.
- Add coconut aminos and fresh basil. Cook for 1 minute more until fluffy.
- Add condiments such as chopped bacon, avocado, coconut flakes, pineapple, scallions, etc.

MAKES TWO (2) SERVINGS

Per serving: 1 serving = 1 cup = 1 vegetable

Mashed Fauxtatoes

One head of cauliflower (or 1 bag of frozen organic roasted cauliflower florets from Trader Joe's®).
Four cloves garlic
1/3-1/2 cup unsweetened almond milk
dash smoked paprika
dash liquid smoke
2 Tsp Kerrygold® butter, melted
sea salt and pepper to taste
coconut oil spray

- Heat oven to 400 degrees
- Remove skin from garlic cloves and place on parchment paper on a cookie sheet for 20-30 minutes
- If using a head of cauliflower, cut into florets and place on a cookie sheet with parchment paper. If you bought the pre-cut pre-roasted bag, then just place florets on the sheet.
- Add the cauliflower to the roasting garlic in the oven.
- Spray cauliflower with oil and roast cauliflower for 30-45 minutes (if fresh), 20-25 minutes (if frozen). Roast until edges are blackened, or cauliflower warms.
- In a food processor, add cauliflower, garlic, almond milk, liquid smoke, and butter.
- Pulse until smooth.

- Serve warm with sprinkles of smoked paprika.

MAKES TWO (2) SERVINGS

Per serving: 1 serving = 1 cup = 1 vegetable

Asparagus with Glaze and Lemon Rind

1 lb fresh asparagus trimmed

1 TBL avocado oil

3 TBL balsamic vinegar

3 TBL Bragg's® aminos or coconut aminos

1 TBL honey

One lemon

*2 Tsp (optional) organic instant coffee crystals

salt and pepper to taste

- Heat grill or grill pan over medium heat.
- Brush asparagus with oil and grill for 3 minutes.
- Turn the asparagus and grill for another 3 minutes.
- In a small saucepan, stir together vinegar, amino acids, honey and coffee crystals (optional). Bring to a boil for 3 minutes until slightly reduced.
- Arrange grilled asparagus on a platter.
- Drizzle the glaze over the asparagus.
- Use the zest of one lemon to sprinkle on top for some extra taste.
- Salt and pepper to taste (optional).

MAKES ONE (1) TO TWO (2) SERVINGS (IF USING THIN SPEARS)

Per serving: 1 serving = 10 asparagus spears = 1 vegetable and 1 Tsp oil/butter

Roasted Coconut Broccoli

One bag frozen broccoli florets (or the head of one broccoli)
Two cloves crushed garlic
Two Tsp red chili flakes
6 TBL unsweetened coconut flakes
1 TBL coconut aminos
2 TBL organic coconut oil
1/4 Tsp salt

- Preheat oven to 375 degrees Fahrenheit.
- In a cast iron skillet (or parchment paper-lined cookie sheet) place the broccoli florets.
- Evenly distribute chili flakes, crush garlic, coconut flakes, and coconut aminos.
- Top with evenly distributed dollops of coconut oil and salt.
- Roast for approximately 20 minutes and stir to re-coat the broccoli.
- Cook for another 20-25 minutes or until the broccoli has crisped and browned edges.

MAKES TWO (2) SERVINGS

Per serving: 1 serving = 1 cup = 1 vegetable

Cauliflower Pizza Crust

2 cups cauliflower, rice frozen (from Trader Joe's®)
1 cup organic grated cheese (cheddar, mozzarella, etc.)
2 eggs
seasoning of choice (like Italian, etc.)
1/4 Tsp salt

▸ Preheat oven to 450 degrees Fahrenheit.
▸ On a cookie sheet lined with parchment paper, lay out the mixture in a nice circle.
▸ Cook crust for 15 minutes or until the crust is golden brown but not burned.

MAKES TWO (2) SERVINGS

Per serving: 1 vegetable, 2 healthful fats, 1/2 protein

Mexican Beef Stew

This household staple is one of my all-time favorites. Inspired by *NomNom Paleo* Braised Beef, I've made a few personal adjustments to fit my family's preferences and tastes. Use fewer liquids, if you wish to use the melt-in-your-mouth beef as a gyro sandwich stuffer. I like to make this in my Instant Pot because I can sauté the onions and add the rest of the ingredients without changing pots—not to mention, the process completes in less than one hour's time. Top it off with fresh guacamole, and you can enjoy a taste of heaven.

3 pounds boneless beef short ribs, beef stew meat or chuck roast cut into 1-inch cubes

2 TBL chili powder

1 Tsp sea salt

1 TBL avocado oil

One large onion chopped

4 TBL tomato paste

Six garlic cloves, peeled and mashed

One jar Roasted Garlic Chipotle Salsa from Trader Joe's®

*1 12 oz can (optional) La Costeña® chipotle pepper in adobo sauce

1/2 cup chicken or beef bone broth

1 and 1/2 Tsp Bragg's® amino acids or Red Boat fish sauce

1/2 cup minced cilantro

Add fresh guacamole for garnish (lime, salt, cilantro, mashed avocado).

- In a large bowl mix the sea salt, chili powder, and meat. Coat well.
- In a separate pan melt oil over medium heat in the oven. If using an InstantPot, then place oil directly in the pot.
- Add onions until translucent.
- Stir in tomato paste and garlic cloves.
- Add seasoned beef, salsa, chipotle peppers, liquid aminos (or fish sauce) and bone broth.
- Push "stew" setting on the InstantPot and walk away or bring ingredients to a boil and either transfer to a crock pock or pressure cooker and cook on stew setting. You can also place the ingredients in an oven-safe Dutch pan at 325 degrees for three hours on the middle rack.
- You will have melt in your mouth beef in less than 45 minutes!

MAKES APPROXIMATELY NINE (9) SERVINGS

Per serving: 1 serving = 1 and 1/2 cups of stew = 1/2 fruit and 1 protein; 1/4 cup of guacamole = 1 healthful fat

Beef Lettuce Wraps

These remind me of the lettuce wraps offered at PF Chang's®. I have created my rendition of an all-time favorite. Not only are these wraps quick and easy, but the flavor profile is incredibly satisfying: spicy, sweet, tangy and salty! You can try ground turkey and chicken if you prefer.

1 TBL toasted sesame oil

1 lb ground grass fed beef (you can find in the frozen section at Trader Joe's®)

1 cup chopped crimini or portabella mushrooms

Four cloves garlic

1 TBL fresh grated ginger root

1/4 cup chopped fresh basil

1/4 cup chopped fresh mint

1/4 cup chopped fresh cilantro

1/2 Tsp red chili pepper flakes

1 TBL Red Boat® fish sauce

1 lime

2 TBL coconut aminos (for sweetness)

1 TBL Bragg's® aminos

salt to taste

One head butter leaf lettuce or artisan romaine lettuce

* 1 TBL of plum sauce

*1/2 cup grated carrot

*1/2 cup chopped water chestnut

*2 TBL chopped green onion

- Heat oil in a skillet over medium high heat.
- Add garlic and chili pepper flakes and cook until the garlic is slightly brown.
- Add the beef and cook until no longer pink.

- Add juice from one lime, fish sauce, and liquid aminos.
- Lastly, add the fresh herbs and salt to taste.
- *Add the optional items if you want a little variety.
- Serve warm in butter leaf lettuce cups, artisan romaine or over-sized cabbage or lettuce leaf.

MAKES APPROXIMATELY FOUR (4) SERVINGS

Per serving: 3/4 cup = 1 protein, 1 Tsp oil/butter, 1 vegetable (1/2 head of butter leaf lettuce)

Turkey Chili

Nothing beats a nice warm bowl of chili on a cold winter's day. If you prefer, you may substitute the ground turkey for ground beef or ground chicken breast.

1 TBL avocado oil
1 lb ground turkey
One medium onion, chopped
One medium bell pepper
Four cloves garlic, finely chopped
1 and 1/2 Tsp cumin
1 Tsp chili powder
1/2 Tsp smoked paprika or chipotle powder
One 6 oz can tomato paste
1 16 oz jar salsa of your choice (I like Trader Joe's® Garlic Chipotle)

1 15 oz can roasted and diced red tomatoes

1 Tsp salt

1/2 cup fresh cilantro

1/4 cup homemade guacamole (mashed avocado, a splash of lime juice, a dash of salt, and 1 1 Tsp of fresh chopped cilantro).

▸ Place all ingredients in a crock pot and cook overnight OR

▸ Heat oil in a sauce pan over medium high heat.

▸ Add turkey, onion, peppers, and garlic; cook until meat is no longer pink.

▸ Add all spices, including salt and cook until aromatic (about 1 minute).

▸ Add salsa, tomato paste, and tomatoes.

▸ Bring to a boil, then put the stove on low and cook for an additional 20 minutes.

▸ Top a bowl of chili off, with 2 TBL of fresh cilantro and homemade guacamole.

MAKES FOUR (4) SERVINGS

Per Serving: 2 cups of chili = 1 protein, 1 fruit, 1 Tsp oil/butter; 1/4 cup guacamole = 1 healthful fat

Quick Smokey Green Chile Chicken

I am usually putting chicken breasts in stock and cooking them in my Instant Pot every day. The Instant Pot creates the perfect pull-apart shredded chicken. Depending on my mood I'll cook the chicken in salsa, chipotle pepper sauce or anything that is leftover in my refrigerator. As an example of a great salad topping, I've included an option for you, using salsa verde.

Two organic chicken breasts
2 cups water or chicken stock
16 oz jar salsa verde
1 Tsp liquid smoke

- In an Instant Pot or Crock Pot, cook the chicken breasts in the chicken stock until the chicken easily pulls apart.
- Place the chicken in a medium sized bowl and mash it with a fork.
- Add in with the salsa verde.
- Add liquid smoke.
- Serve mixture in a seaweed wrap, a grain-free soft tortilla shell OR Gyro Sandwich Wraps (see the recipe for Pizza Crust).
- Top with fresh cilantro and homemade guacamole (1/4 cup).

MAKES FOUR (4) SERVINGS

Per serving: 1 protein, 1 vegetable

Chicken Salad

Four organic chicken breasts

1/2 packet organic onion soup mix

3/4 cup Homemade Mayonnaise (see recipe)

1/2 cup chopped pickles

1/2 cup chopped celery

1/2 cup chopped cilantro

2 TBL freshly chopped chives

1 TBL fresh dill

freshly cracked pepper

* 2 Tsp Dijon-like mustard (optional)

2 cups water or chicken stock

- In an Instant Pot or Crock Pot, cook the chicken breasts in the chicken stock until the chicken easily pulls apart.
- Place the chicken in a medium sized bowl and mash it with a fork.
- Add in all of the other ingredients.
- Serve mixture in a seaweed wrap, a grain-free soft tortilla shell OR Gyro Sandwich Wraps (see the recipe for Pizza Crust) or top 1/4 of the mixture over mixed greens for a fantastic salad.
- Top with fresh cilantro and homemade guacamole

MAKES FOUR (4) SERVINGS

Per serving: 1 protein, 1.5 oil/butter

Buffalo Chicken

Four organic chicken breasts

1/2 cup Kerrygold® butter or coconut oil

4 TBL Frank's® hot sauce

*1 Tsp liquid smoke (optional)

- In an Instant Pot or Crock Pot, cook the chicken breasts in the chicken stock until the chicken easily pulls apart.
- Place the chicken in a medium sized bowl and mash it with a fork.
- Add in all of the other ingredients.
- Serve mixture mixed with shredded cabbage and top with homemade guacamole!!! You can even create some buffalo tacos by using the sandwich wrap recipe in Complex Carbohydrates or try the savory version of the Almond Flour Pancakes.

MAKES FOUR (4) SERVINGS

Per serving: 1 protein, 2 oil/butter

Chicken Kale Soup (with Bacon Fat: optional)

I can't describe the amount of inner warmth that a good bowl of soup can provide. Thankfully, this soup is not only nourishing but incredibly delicious. It is easy to make enough for leftovers if you wish to make some in bulk.

Two organic chicken breasts

4 cups chicken broth (homemade chicken bone broth is ideal)

3-4 cups of baby kale

1/2 sweet onion, chopped

Six garlic cloves, mashed with a fork

One sweet red pepper, chopped

4 TBL of bacon fat (from 1lb of applewood smoked bacon)

1/2 Tsp sea salt

1/4 Tsp ground black pepper

1/2 Tsp Trader Joe's® 21 Seasoning Salute (or Spike®)

10-12 fresh basil leaves

*1 Tsp liquid smoke (if no bacon fat)

*1 cup carrots, chopped (optional)

*1 cup celery, chopped (optional)

- In an Instant Pot or Crock Pot, cook the chicken breasts in the chicken stock until the chicken easily pulls apart.
- Preheat oven to 375 degrees. Place the bacon on parchment paper, in a pan or cookie tray. Once the oven is heated, cook the bacon for 17-20 minutes until browned and slightly crispy. Drain off the bacon fat into a glass container and store excess in the refrigerator for seasoning foods.
- Cut bacon into 1/4 inch pieces and add to the soup.
- Place the chicken in a medium sized bowl and mash it with a fork.

- Add in all of the other ingredients.
- Serve warm.

MAKES FOUR (4) SERVINGS

Per serving: 1 protein, 1 vegetable, 1 oil/butter

Chicken Bone Broth

There is no better way to nourish your gut (and your body) than to drink bone broth. The anti-inflammatory, gut healing, immune boosting, brain boosting, collagen-producing, anti-aging, detoxification, etc. benefits are too numerous to count. If you have ever ventured to make your bone broth, then you know that it is easy to make and it tastes SO good, you will want to drink it out of a mug. In fact, I often do.

Two organic chicken carcasses (I save the bones from two rotisserie chickens), broken up, so they fit in your Crock Pot or Instant Pot.
8 cups of filtered water
Two medium leeks, sliced into coin-size pieces or one large onion, sliced
One large carrot, sliced into coin size pieces
Four stalks of celery, chopped
Six garlic cloves, mashed with a fork
2-inch piece of ginger root, sliced into coin size pieces
1 TBL Red Boat® fish sauce

1 TBL Bragg's® apple cider vinegar

Two chicken feet (NOTE: if you can get chicken feet from your local farmer or your Asian market, add two chicken feet into the pot. Chicken feet will create a remarkable gelatinous effect that will be super tasty when heated (and provide even more nutrition for you).

*2 bay leaves (optional)

- Put all of your ingredients in an eight-quart slow cooker or pressure cooker. If needed, add in filtered water so that all of the bones are submerged. Make sure that you have ready any precautionary instructions for your cooking vessel to ensure that you have not overfilled.

- If using your Instant Pot, elect soup butter and set the pressure to "low" and increase the cook time to 120 minutes. After the two hours have completed, allow the cooker to depressurize naturally by not releasing the valve. Strain the broth and discard the bones and vegetables. Pour the broth into mason jars and store in your refrigerator.

- If using a Crock Pot, cover and cook on low for 8-24 hours. The longer, the better. Strain the broth and discard the bones and vegetables. Pour the broth into mason jars and store in your refrigerator.

- When you are ready, drink the broth after reheating on the stove to liquify the gelatin. Enjoy!

MAKES EIGHT (8) SERVINGS

Crab Cakes (or Salmon Cakes)

1 and 1/2 pounds canned boneless, skinless wild salmon or crab

1/4 cup Homemade Mayonnaise or avocado mayonnaise

2 TBL ghee

2 large eggs

Two scallions, thinly sliced

1/4 cup diced red bell pepper

1/2 cup chopped yellow onion

Two cloves garlic minced

Two tsp Old Bay Seasoning®

1 TBL tapioca starch

1 TBL freshly chopped Italian parsley

1 Tsp smoked paprika

1/2 Tsp Himalayan salt

1/4 Tsp white pepper

1/2 Tsp Dijon-like mustard

▸ In a large bowl mix the fish, mayo, eggs, parsley, onion, tapioca flour, smoked paprika, Old Bay Seasoning, salt, dijon mustard, minced garlic and white pepper.

▸ Once you have divided the mixture into eight equal parts, form each part into a patty, roughly 3 inches in diameter and 3/4 inch thick.

- Place patties in the refrigerator while you mix the breading and make the aïoli.
- After you have mixed the breading mixture and prepared the aïoli, you are ready to heat the stove.
- Heat the ghee over medium heat in a large cast-iron skillet.
- Lightly coat each patty with the breading mixture, making sure to shake off excess flour.
- Once the ghee has melted and coated the pan, you may fry the cakes for 2 minutes on each side until golden brown.
- Serve warm with lemon wedges and Italian parsley.
- Top with the aïoli.

Breading

1/4 cup coconut flour

1/4 cup tapioca flour

1 TBLOld Bay Seasoning®

Smoked Aïoli

1 cup Homemade Mayonnaise

2 TBL Dijon-style mustard

1 TBL capers, finely chopped

Two tsp fresh lemon juice

1 Tsp freshly minced garlic clove

1 Tsp smoked paprika

splash liquid smoke

1/4 Tsp Himalayan sea salt

▸ Mix all ingredients in a food processor.
▸ Store excess in the refrigerator for five days.

MAKES EIGHT (8) CAKES OR FOUR (4) SERVINGS

Per serving: 2 cakes = 1 protein, 1 seed/dressings, 1 oil/butter, 1/4 complex carb

A serving size = 2 tablespoons (TBL).

Guacamole dressing

Two medium avocados, ripened, pitted and peeled.

1 cup freshly chopped cilantro

Two limes, juiced

1/2 cup avocado oil

1/2 Tsp red chili pepper flakes

salt and pepper to taste

- Mix all ingredients in a food processor until smooth.
- Store in a 2 cup mason jar in the refrigerator.
- Use the dressing quickly before it turns brown.

Vinaigrette

8 TBL extra virgin olive oil or avocado oil

1/2 lemon freshly juiced fresh lemon juice

6 drops liquid stevia

1/2 TBL Dijon-like mustard

8 TBL balsamic vinegar

- In a small bowl, mix all ingredients with a fork or whisk. Store in a mason jar in the refrigerator.

Citrus Mint Dressing

1/4 cup fresh lime juice

1/4 cup fresh grapefruit or orange juice

1/2 cup freshly chopped mint leaves

6 drops liquid stevia

1/4 cup avocado oil

1/4 Tsp Himalayan salt

white pepper to taste

- Mix all ingredients in a food processor.
- Store in a mason jar in the refrigerator.

Creamy Asian Spicy Dressing

1/4 cup coconut aminos

Six fresh basil leaves

3 TBL Homemade Mayonnaise

3 TBL toasted sesame oil

Two Tsp Trader Joe's® Spicy Jalepeño Sauce

1/4 Tsp Himalayan salt to taste

- Mix all ingredients in a food processor.

▸ Store in a mason jar in the refrigerator.

Smokey BBQ sauce

16 oz can or jar tomato sauce

4 TBL tomato paste

1/2 cup Bragg's® apple cider vinegar

5 TBL raw honey or my preference is "Simple Syrup" made from xylitol (see recipe)

1/2 TBL ground black pepper

1/2 TBL onion powder

1/2 TBL ground mustard

One Tsp smoked paprika

1 TBL lemon juice

1/2 Tsp liquid smoke

1/2 to 3/4 cup water

*1/2 Tsp (optional) chipotle powder

*2 Tsp Trader Joe's® Jalepeño Hot Sauce or 1 Tsp of cayenne pepper

▸ In a medium sized sauce pan, heat all ingredients, except the water and liquid smoke).

▸ Bring ingredients to a boil, then let sit.

▸ After 30 minutes, assess the thickness. If it is too thick, add 1/4-1/2 cup of water and reheat, then let sit for another 30 minutes.

▸ Add the liquid smoke and any optional flavors that you wish.

- Add any additional water until it is the desired consistency or leave as thick as you wish.
- Store in an air-tight container in your refrigerator.

Vegan Peanut Sauce

One lime juiced

Two Tsp finely grated ginger

2/3 cup organic creamy peanut butter

1 TBL Hoisen sauce

2 TBL spicy Thai chile sauce or Sriracha

1 TBL coconut aminos

1 TBL Bragg's® amino acids

1/2 cup full-fat coconut milk

1/2 cup water

- Bring all ingredients to a medium heat temperature.
- Whisk until peanut butter is smooth.
- Slowly add water or coconut milk up to 1 cup, to achieve the desired consistency.

Ketchup

7 oz can tomato paste

2 TBL Bragg's® apple cider vinegar

One scoop stevia powder or 8 drops of liquid

1/2 Tsp Himalayan sea salt

1/2 Tsp garlic powder

1/2 Tsp onion powder

1/4 Tsp allspice

1/2 TBL molasses or yacon syrup (for low glycemic sweetness that builds bones)

1/4 cup filtered water

*1/8 Tsp (optional) cayenne

- Heat all ingredients over medium heat (do NOT boil).
- Once warm, remove from the stove and let sit until room temp.
- Refrigerate in an air-tight container.

Homemade Mayonnaise

Three large egg yolks (room temperature)

1/2 Tsp Himalayan salt

1/4 Tsp Dijon-style mustard

1/2 TBL white vinegar or champagne vinegar

12 TBL freshly squeezed lemon

One and 1/2-2 cups avocado or macadamia nut oil.

- Fill a blender with boiling water and let sit for a few minutes.
- Pour out the water and lightly dry the inside with a towel.
- On medium speed, mix the egg yolks until thick.
- Add the salt and mustard, quickly.
- Add the vinegar and lemon juice and pulse until well blended.

- With the motor running on low speed, begin adding the oil and the slowest speed you can pour.
- Half way through, the mayonnaise should appear like thick cream.
- You can now add the rest of the oil. Be careful not to pour too fast as the mixture may curdle.
- Once all of the oil is added, and the mixture seems a bit too thick, just add a smidge of vinegar or lemon to smooth it out.
- Store the mayo in an air-tight container in the refrigerator for up to 5 days

Apple Pie Alkalizing Water

24 oz to 32 oz water in a water bottle or mason jar

3 TBL Bragg's® Apple Cider Vinegar

2 TBL freshly squeezed lemon juice

6-8 drops liquid stevia

2 shakes cinnamon or pumpkin pie spice

‣ Add all ingredients to a water bottle, to go cup or mason jar.

‣ Enjoy your extremely healthy water and drink as much as you like.

Lemonade Water

24 oz to 32 oz water in a water bottle or mason jar

2 TBL freshly squeezed lemon juice

6-8 drops liquid stevia

‣ Add all ingredients to a water bottle, to go cup or mason jar.

‣ Enjoy your extremely healthy water and drink as much as you like.

Fauxjito

8 oz carbonated water or club soda

10 fresh mint leaves

1/2 lime juiced

1/2 lime garnish

1 cup ice cubes

2 TBL sugar-free simple syrup

- Muddle the mint and lime garnish in the glass.
- Add the simple syrup and ice.
- Fill the glass with carbonated water.

Cucumber and Lime Water

24 oz to 32 oz water in a water bottle or mason jar

2 TBL freshly squeezed lime juice

6-8 muddled fresh mint

1/2 cup sliced cucumber

- Add all ingredients to a water bottle, to go cup or mason jar.
- Enjoy your extremely healthy water and drink as much as you like.

Cranberry Cleanse Water

Cranberry Cleanse Water is a great concoction for treating cellulite, aiding bladder infections, providing a natural diuresis-like activity for the kidneys and overall detoxification.

28 oz water in a 30 oz water bottle or mason jar

4 oz unsweetened cranberry juice

2 TBL freshly squeezed lemon juice

6-8 drops stevia liquid

***2-4 bags (optional) decaffeinated chai tea for spice**

- Add all ingredients to a water bottle, to go cup or mason jar.
- Enjoy your extremely healthy water and drink as much as you like.

Plantain Cinnamon Faux-nuts *

These lovely safe-carb desserts are perfect for those times you crave something sweet and bread-like but need to stay on track. Consider this fun treat a great transition into a no grain diet.

One ripe plantain (make sure it is black on the outside and soft to

the touch)

1-1 and 1/2 cups tapioca flour

1 egg

1 cup virgin or unrefined coconut oil

One Tsp cinnamon

1/2 Tsp vanilla

*1 cup of roasted apple, chopped

sea salt to taste

▸ Heat oil in a small saucepan.

▸ You want the oil to melt to at least one (1) inch in depth.

▸ With your hands, mash up the plantain in a bowl. Add the vanilla and egg. It will be a messy process, FYI.

▸ Add 1/4 of the tapioca flour and mix thoroughly.

▸ Continue to add 1/4 of the flour until you have the consistency of pizza dough (you may need more or less flour, depending on your consistency).

- Roll out the dough with a rolling pin on a cutting board dusted with tapioca flour.
- Roll to about a 1/4 inch thickness.
- With a drinking glass or lid with a 2-3 inch diameter opening, cut out perfect circles of dough.
- When the oil is sufficiently heated, use a slotted spoon to drop a few doughnuts in gently.
- Cook evenly about 1-2 minutes per side or until golden brown.
- With your slotted spoon, remove the doughnut and place on a paper towel-covered plate.
- Sprinkle with cinnamon and sea salt.
- Serve warm.
- * If you want to make an "apple fritter," roast a Fuji, Gala or Granny Smith apple ahead of time. Remove the core of the apple, slice the apple and place in the oven at 375 degrees until soft (approximately 25 minutes). Chop up the slices into smaller pieces and add the apple bits into your dough.

MAKES FOUR (4) SERVINGS

Per serving: 3-4 faux-nuts = 1 complex carb and approximately 1 oil

Chocolate Truffles

12 oz stevia-sweetened dark chocolate (Lily's® or Coco Polo®). These bars are a bit pricey so if you are on a budget, Trader

Joe's® makes a nice one: the Dark Chocolate Lover's Chocolate Bar (85% cacao); however, these bars are not free of sugar. Shave the chocolate bars into small shavings with a sharp knife.

3 TBL coconut butter

1 cup Trader Joe's® coconut cream (or the cream from a full-fat coconut milk can that has been chilled to consolidate the cream and separate it from the liquid).

1 and 1/2 Tsp vanilla extract

1/2 Tsp sea salt

Other items you may choose to add into your truffles:

*1/4 cup ground hazelnuts (optional flavor choice)

*1 Tsp of instant coffee (optional flavor choice)

*1/4 cup PB Fit® peanut butter powder + 3 TBL of water

*1 and 1/2 TBL raw maca powder (superfood choice)

*2 Tsp Mucuna pruriens powder (superfood choice)

Topping for Truffles

1/2 cup topping of choice (see options below and mix and match if you are crazy like that):

*raw cacao (my favorite)

*slightly toasted unsweetened shredded coconut flakes

*1 Tsp cinnamon

▸ Heat coconut cream in a small sauce pan over low heat.

- Put shaved chocolate and coconut butter into a medium-sized mixing bowl.
- Pour the melted coconut cream over the chocolate shavings and coconut cream and stir very gently until the mixture is uniform in color.
- Add vanilla, sea salt and any of the optional flavorings or superfoods that you choose (*). If you are using hazelnuts, add them now.
- Put the bowl into the refrigerator for 1-2 hours until the mixture firms up, and you can spoon out 1-2 tablespoons at a time.
- Once the truffle dough is chilled, let the mixture stand at room temperature for 30 minutes before coating. Spoon out 1-2 tablespoons at a time and form balls. Roll each ball in your mixture of choice (toasted coconut or raw cacao).
- Place each ball on a parchment paper lined cookie sheet and chill for 4-5 hours.
- These truffles can be put in the freezer to keep or kept in the refrigerator for two weeks, in an airtight container.

MAKES TWELVE SERVINGS

Per serving: 1 cheat

Flourless Chocolate "Cake"

This recipe might as well be called "Lovers Cake." This one wins out for Valentine's Day and special occasions with a loved one, every time. Make sure you have some fun red wine and your favorite "mood" music in the background when you serve this. If the evening ends well, I have warned you fairly. You're welcome!

7 oz stevia-sweetened dark chocolate (Lily's® or Coco Polo®). These bars are a bit pricey so if you are on a budget, Trader Joe's® makes a nice dark chocolate bar: the Dark Chocolate Lover's Chocolate Bar (85% cacao); however, these bars are *not* free of sugar but are low in sugar. Shave the chocolate bars into small shavings with a sharp knife.
One can Trader Joe's® coconut cream + 1 can for topping
Two egg yolks
1/8 Tsp sea salt
1/4 Tsp chili powder
1/4 Tsp cardamom powder
1/4 Tsp cinnamon
1 TBL vanilla

- Refrigerate your coconut cream so that the cream and coconut water separate.
- Use a sharp knife to chop the chocolate into small shavings. Put all of the shavings into a bowl.
- Put the coconut cream (*no coconut water from the can*), two egg yolks, salt, chili powder, cardamom powder and cinnamon in a medium-sized sauce pan.
- Whisk together in a sauce pan over low heat. Do not leave it alone. Watch it closely *making sure it doesn't boil* or overheat. Keep stirring with a whisk over low heat for approximately 10 minutes until the custard sticks to the back of a wooden spoon.

- When the custard has stuck to the back of a spoon, it is ready to take off of the stove.
- Pour the liquid custard over a netted fine mesh sieve, positioned over the chocolate shavings.
- Add the 1 TBL of vanilla.
- Let the chocolate and warm custard sit for 5 minutes.
- Spray four ramekins with some coconut oil spray.
- When the chocolate mixture has sat for 5 minutes, then gently FOLD, *slowly* with a spatula.
- Pour the chocolate loveliness into four small ramekins.
- Let the filled ramekins sit for 30 minutes.
- Refrigerate for 4 hours.
- You can turn the ramekins upside down and pop the cakes onto a beautiful serving plate. Let sit at room temperature for at least an hour for the ideal consistency for eating.
- **FOR TOPPING:** Take the refrigerated coconut cream from the second can. Whip in 1 Tsp of vanilla extract, 1/8 Tsp of cardamom powder and about four drops of liquid stevia.

MAKES EIGHT (8) SERVINGS, FOUR (4) RAMEKINS

Per serving: 1 cheat

Peanut Butter Chocolate Truffles

3 TBL PB Fit® powder or any peanut powder (PB and Me®, PB2®, etc.)

1 TBL raw cacao

2 1/2 TBL xylitol mixed with 2 1/2 TBL of boiling water, until no granules are visible.

2 TBL coconut butter

2 shakes sea salt

1/4 cup unsweetened coconut flakes

1/2 Tsp vanilla

- ▸ Mix all ingredients.
- ▸ Scoop out rounded tablespoons into balls and rolling a mixture of coconut flakes and raw cacao.
- ▸ Put in the fridge for 30 minutes to 1 hour.

MAKES FOUR (4) SERVINGS

Per serving: 1 cheat

Keto Coconut Bars

These Coconut Bars are some of my favorite "fat bombs" when I need something on the go to provide energy and nourishment during the day. Who needs it for dessert when you can have it for breakfast?

2 cups coconut oil, melted

1 cup unsweetened coconut flakes (toasted for 2-5 minutes)

1 cup macadamia nuts, chopped fine in a food processor

1/2 cup chia seeds

1/2 cup hemp seeds

Two Tsp vanilla

3 TBL xylitol

2 shakes sea salt

- ▸ Mix all ingredients.
- ▸ In an 8 inch by 8-inch pyrex dish, lined with parchment paper, pour in the mixture. Put the mixture in the freezer.
- ▸ Serve when the mixture has fully hardened (about 1 hour).

MAKES EIGHT (8) SERVINGS

Per serving: 4 oils, 2 nut/seed

Coconut Collagen and Cacao Nib Bites

1 cup almond flour

1/4 cup unsweetened coconut flakes (finely shredded)

1/4 cup coconut oil

2 TBL coconut sugar

2 TBL almond butter

2 TBL Great Lakes Collagen®

2 TBL cacao nibs

1 Tsp vanilla

2 shakes sea salt

1/4 Tsp cinnamon

- Mix all ingredients.
- Scoop out rounded tablespoons into balls and roll the balls in shredded coconut flakes.
- Put in the fridge for 5-10 minutes.

MAKES FOUR (4) SERVINGS

Per serving: 1 complex carb, 2 oil/butter

Sweet Potato & Pumpkin Crustless Pie *

This pie recipe is one of my favorite treats that I allow myself on special occasions, like Thanksgiving or even as my once per week treat, if I feel the love.

One can pumpkin purée (not pumpkin pie filling)

2 cups roasted Muraski sweet potatoes (Trader Joe's®), mashed. You can use regular sweet potato if you can't find the Murasaki type. Just make sure it is not a yam. Look for cream colored inside, not orange.

3/4 cup full-fat coconut milk

1/3 cup xylitol, melted into 1/3 cup of boiling water

3 TBL almond flour

Two egg yolks

Two whole eggs

1 TBL vanilla extract (in alcohol, not glycerine)

1/2 Tsp sea salt

1 and 1/2 Tsp pumpkin pie spice

One Tsp cardamom

1 12 Tsp ground ginger or freshly grated ginger

1/2 Tsp clove

One Tsp nutmeg (ideally, freshly grated)

One Tsp cinnamon

- Preheat oven to 350 degrees.
- Spray an 8 inch by 8-inch pyrex dish with coconut oil spray.
- Place 1/2 inch of water in a larger dish in which to set your 8x8 pyrex pan.
- Mix all ingredients with a mixer until smooth.
- Cook for approximately 50 minutes or until a fork comes out clean.
- Let cool at room temperature or serve hot, topped with coconut cream topping (see flourless chocolate cake).

MAKES EIGHT (8) SERVINGS

Per serving: 1 complex carb

SNACK IDEAS:

- Two hard-boiled eggs

  Per Serving: 1 protein

- 24 almonds and one pear

  Per Serving: 1 healthful fat, 1 fruit

- 2 TBL of roasted pumpkin seeds and one apple

  Per Serving: 1 healthy fat, 1 fruit

- One roasted sweet potato with 2 TBL of almond butter or 1 TBL of Kerryygold® butter

  Per Serving: 1 complex carb, 1 butter

- 2 pre-made egg muffins

  Per Serving: 1 protein, 1 vegetable

- 3/4 cup of full-fat cottage cheese, 4 TBL toasted, sliced almonds, 2 TBL unsweetened dried berries

  Per Serving: 1 protein, 1 nut/seeds

- 3/4 cup unsweetened, organic Greek yogurt (full-fat), 3/4 cup blackberries, 4 TBL sliced almonds or 2 TBL hemp seeds

  Per Serving: 1 protein, 1 fruit, 1 nut/seeds

- FUN CHEAT: 10 fancy olives, 4 TBL or 1 oz of artisan cheese, 12 roasted almonds, 1/2 sliced pear, 1 oz of 85% dark chocolate, 5 oz wine

  Per Serving: 1 healthful fat, 1/2 fruit, 2 cheats. This cheat is fun on a no complex carbohydrate day.

- Devil's Food Cake flavored Paleo Protein Bar by Julien Bakery®

  Per Serving: 1 protein, 1/2 of fat, one complex carb

- 4 oz Applegate® turkey breast slices wrapped up in romaine lettuce leaves with 1/4 avocado sliced, and one red pepper cut lengthwise topped with 2 TBL of homemade mayonnaise. Make lettuce wraps.

  Per Serving: 1 protein, 1 vegetable, 1 healthful fat, 1 oil

- High-protein low-carb dark chocolate almond bar by Primal Kitchen®

  Per Serving: 1 protein, 1/2 complex carb, and 1 fat

NOT-SO-NAUGHTY NIGHT CAPS

These fun cocktails are considered a "CHEAT" so make sure you are monitoring your complex carbohydrate and fruit intake for the day if you choose to imbibe. If you need a reference, review **The Plan: Calculate Your Calories**.

TIP:

*Limit your total servings of red wine or cocktails to six per week. If you decide to have a cocktail, include the drink in your total servings of cheats for the week. If you want to lose weight, I suggest **no more than three** servings of wine or alcohol per week (ideally on the same day). If you are sensitive to sulfites, try wines from Heartswork Winery, such as Well Red or try Roule Rouge (you can purchase both at Trader Joe's) as neither wine has added sulfites and are certified low in sulfites. A paleo friendly wine acclaimed for being free of headaches and hangovers is Dry Farms Wines. You can purchase both reds and whites (and bubbly) from their web page dryfarmwines.com. Fit Vine Wines produce my new favorite. They don't use pesticides, use advanced filtration, and their wine has no residual sugars. As a bonus, each 5 oz glass only has 95 calories. With about $16 plus shipping, you can get a fabulous bottle of wine delivered to your door from fitvinewines.com*

Sugar-Free Simple Syrup

You can enjoy simple syrup several ways, depending on your preference (Xylitol or Truvia are my preferences. Keep a mason jar loaded in your refrigerator of pre-made syrup so that in a pinch, you can prepare a fun drink for you and your loved ones.

Xylitol Simple Syrup

1 cup hot water (not boiling)
1 cup Xylitol

- Mix the two ingredients until the xylitol dissolves entirely in the solution.
- Cool at room temperature and store in an airtight container in the refrigerator.

Truvia® Simple Syrup

4 TBL Truvia® spoonable stevia or 12 packets
1/2 cup warm water

- Mix the two ingredients until the Truvia® dissolves entirely in the solution.
- Cool at room temperature and store in an airtight container in the refrigerator.

Stevia Simple Syrup

1/4 cup stevia powder (or approximately 20 packets)
2 cups warm water

- Mix the two ingredients until the stevia dissolves entirely in the solution.
- Cool at room temperature and store in an airtight container in the refrigerator.

Dramfauxie (similar to Drambuie)

1 pint Indio Spirits® James Oliver Bourbon Barreled American Whiskey (very smooth) or Granddad® Bourbon Whiskey or your favorite Scotch whiskey.
2 TBL licorice root
4 TBL simple syrup made from xylitol (see recipe below)
Two Tsp honey powder OR 2 droppers-full of honey flavored extract

- For 24-72 hours, infuse the bourbon with the anise seeds or licorice root.
- Once you have infused the bourbon, use a strainer to filter the seeds from the liquid.

- Add the simple xylitol syrup slowly to taste, depending on your taste.
- Add the honey powder or honey-flavored extract to taste (be careful that you don't add it all at once as it may be too sweet for your liking.
- Serve 2-4 ounces of the mixture in a glass over shaved ice or cocktail ice cubes.

French 75

2 oz Indio Spirits® Cricket Club Gin (I like that it has herbal and citrus notes, not juniper)
4-6 oz dry champagne or dry sparkling white wine
1 TBL fresh lemon juice
1 TBL sugar-free simple syrup (see recipe)

- Mix the gin, lemon juice and simple syrup in a cocktail mixer with ice.
- Pour the mixture into a wine glass.
- Add champagne to the mix.
- Garnish with a fresh sage leaf and lemon rind swirl.

NoSweetJo (Mojito Without Sugar)

Two oz Indio Spirits® lime vodka (can you tell I am partial to Indio Spirits?) or white rum

4 oz carbonated water or club soda

10 fresh mint leaves

1/2 lime juiced

1/2 lime garnish

1 cup ice cubes

2 TBL sugar-free simple syrup

‣ Muddle the mint and lime garnish in the glass.

‣ Add the simple syrup and ice.

‣ Fill the glass with carbonated water. Top with the white rum or lime vodka.

MAKES ONE (1) SERVING

Appendix
Printable and Supplemental Materials

You can find all of the printable and supplemental materials you will need to support your success at journeytowardjoy.com. Click on the Resources tab, and you will find the documents mentioned in this book. I have added a quick summary of the worksheets and lists available for your convenience. I suggest that you print them off and use them regularly and as often as you wish.

To work through the affirmation process, print off both **Affirmation Worksheet A** and **Affirmation Worksheet B**. Use Worksheet A to make a list of things you want to change about your body on the left-hand side. Make a list of the ideal version of this trait, on the right-hand side. Be thorough. Once you have your ideals, you can create affirmations surrounding each positive quality. If you need examples, refer to chapter 3. Remember, keep each statement in the present tense and only use positive words.

To prepare for tracking your daily caloric needs and serving amounts, print off the attached chart (**Meal and Serving Tracker**). Write your caloric goal on the sheet and add the recommended servings for each category (using your caloric requirements and suggested servings located on the blue chart in chapter 9). Keep the meal and serving tracker sheet on your refrigerator or take it with you in your purse or briefcase to easily track your eating habits to stay on target. The chart lists the serving size at the top as a reminder; but, remember some foods vary and are different than the measurements listed (i.e., banana, nuts, eggs, apricots, etc.) so always refer to the serving size of each food item if you aren't sure. I suggest that you print enough of the Meal and Serving Tracker sheets for one to two weeks.

If you are the type of person who wishes to track your macros for each meal (again this is not recommended unless you are the kind of person who benefits from micromanagement of your food), then you can use the My Fitness Pal or Cronometer phone application, the **Macronutrient Calculation Worksheets.** Once you figure out your carbohydrates, protein and fat for each meal and you have created a meal plan based on these numbers, you can use the **Meal and Serving Tracker** to keep yourself accountable.

Use the **Workout Planner** to plan a month or two of your workouts. You can start with the primary recommendation provided in chapter 10. The plan as outlined in this chapter is a great place for anyone to begin. Make sure that at a minimum, every three to four weeks, you change things up and add a new exercise, heavier weights, more HIIT, etc. Make sure you are challenging yourself. Phoning it in, will not get you the results you desire. As aforementioned in chapter 11, if you wish to individualize your program even further, you can create a plan based on your body type.

I have attached a thorough **Shopping List** for you to use as a reference. By no means is this list all inclusive. Feel free to add foods that you wish to have (please consider the Approved Foods list, first). Keep this list hung on your refrigerator. When menu planning for the week you can quickly determine what foods to purchase for the week. Mark the "need to get" box to identify your new list for the next grocery run.

If you wish to determine any foods that may be hindering your success or causing water retention and "false fat" from inflammation, then use the **Progress Tracker or the Food and Reaction Tracker.** If you wish to track your weekly progress with measurements to ascertain that you are heading in the right direction with your nutrition and fitness, then use the **Weekly Tracker.** Don't forget that at the end of this book in the **Resources**, you'll find a list of smart phone applications that I use to track fat percentage, BMI, food intake, macronutrients, etc.

About the Author

The journey toward joy in my life has been a culmination of events that provide insight into who I am and how I choose to make a difference in this world. This biography is a summary of those events that have led me to you. It is my intention, in writing this, to paint a picture of my journey thus far. My journey started in grade school.

A childhood pass-time of mine was providing a local hospital for stray animals and injured birds. It was quite common for me to bring home an unfortunate creature, attempt to nurse it back to health in the shoebox hospital and expect miracles. Surprisingly, miracles did occur from time to time, and some of my most pleasurable memories stem from the pets that stuck around after their discharge from my ER.

Around this period, in the throws of grade school, I "published" my first book for a young writers competition. And while "The Bears Downstairs" never made it as a New York Times Best Seller, the process of creating a book stirred a new interest in me that—unbeknownst to me, would blossom much later in life.

In addition to my creation of the Linder Hospital for Animals and The Bears Downstairs, I was obsessed with Teen Magazine and Seventeen Magazine. I couldn't get enough of the fashion and beauty tips. I scoured every page, cover to cover looking for any elixir that might transport me to the likeness of my celebrity idols.

Fast forward a few years to my college years at Northwest University. I continued to foster my interest in the sciences and pursued a degree in biology, graduating magna cum laude. I finally knew that I wanted to be a naturopathic physician and assist people with their health goals. Ironically, to pay for college, a significant portion of my twenties was spent working for many major cosmetic companies, in the realm of makeup artistry and skin care. What I didn't realize was that someday, my passions for natural medicine and aesthetics would collide and form a perfect culminations in a future career.

As I transitioned into the life of a medical student, I began to dive into physiology and biochemistry—and although incredibly challenging for me, science began to provide explanations to many questions I had about weight loss and fat metabolism. While I was never extremely overweight, the desire to be in better shape and lose the extra weight that clung to me since puberty, was always at the forefront of my mind.

After graduating medical school, I accepted the opportunity to teach and direct a pharmacy technician program at a college in Oregon. While it was not practicing medicine, it was teaching within the medical field, requiring continual research of both medical science and education philosophy. I did not know that teaching would soon rise to the top of my list of interests; but, it soon became something that felt "natural" (although my former students may disagree). Quickly, I moved up the ranks and accepted a new position as Director of Education. A couple of years later, I accepted a Dean position of another college, where I continued to teach and develop curriculum. It was in this new position as Dean that I thrived under the mentorship of the Campus President and learned and developed skills in leadership, public speaking, curriculum development, etc. It was my experience as a Dean that sparked a revival of my love for writing which was a distant memory. While the authorship of policies and procedures, accreditation reports and submissions to the State may seem mundane, I thoroughly enjoyed the process of creating and contributing to my community.

In addition to these skills, I welcomed mentorship, training, and certification in high-performance methods using the latest in cognitive psychology and neuroscience. Soon, I created curriculum and instructor training rooted in these concepts that caught the eye of State officials. The insight, leadership, and mentorship I received as a result of this experience remain a pinnacle point in my insatiable hunger and fervent desire to pursue excellence in every area of my life.

As an educator and leader, I grew in my understanding of the importance of research and forever being "the student." To better myself, I began using these skills to soak up everything I could get my hands on for fat loss and fitness. Over time, my application of the research provided a fruitful outcome, and the weight finally came off (ending with a total of 45 pounds lost). I became so passionate about my experience and my transformation that I created a blog post and began writing my first book to assist my friends and family on their journey toward health as well.

During my last years as a Dean — and after many futile attempts at love — I finally met my wonderful husband, John. His support, love and continual encouragement have become the foundation for my joy and freedom to be who I am designed to be.

Soon after our engagement, it was clear that moving both of us into my one bedroom apartment would be a clutter challenge. Given my research skills, I scoured the internet for philosophies, ideas, and motivation for clearing clutter and simplifying our soon-to-be-life, together. Over the process of a year, I developed habits and methods for decluttering and organizing every nook and cranny of our apartment and so by the time we were married, our humble abode was a Martha Stewart Masterpiece (at least that is how I wish to think of it). The joy I created from this pursuit was over-whelming—and as a result, I dedicated myself to helping my friends and family achieve the same enjoyment from always being able to find their keys, amongst every other material item that is important.

After almost ten years in education and management, I felt a strong stirring in my soul to get back to medicine and to begin serving my community in a new way. Around this time, a dear friend and col-league of mine opened a medical facility soon to be on its way to-ward becoming a new and thriving hot spot in Portland, Oregon. After receiving the invitation to come join her in her business, I could not say "no." After all, this new experience was the culmina-tion of my passions: medicine, aesthetics, weight loss and assisting in the occasional blog post; thus providing an avenue to share my talents with Portland. Given the flexibility of my new schedule, I still had time to write and create as part of my desire to serve others, sharing knowledge and assisting my readers with lifestyle challenges. And of course, I continue to find ways I can utilize my organizing and decluttering expertise.

The greatest part of my new career (apart from working with individuals that I love and respect dearly) is that I have the opportunity to serve my community and to make a difference sharing my passions—and what I continue to learn—as a Lifestyle, Health, Wellness and Aging-Well Expert. And naturally, I continue to apply these skills utilizing education as part of the Hippocratic oath: doctor as teacher.

My medical philosophy is that optimum health and well-being encompasses every aspect of one's life. The many dimensions to investigate include one's endeavor toward spiritual growth; pursuing one's passions; physically challenging fitness activity; consuming proper nutrition; building healthy relationships; serving others and strategically simplifying one's life to make room for these critical components of a fulfilling existence. In essence, I believe that holistic medicine expands well beyond nutrition, supplements, medications, and modalities. And how does my passion for aesthetics fit in with this philosophy, you ask? In my opinion, people are the most beautiful when they understand—and are pursuing— their utmost potential, in the areas listed above. The tools we use in the clinic — while seemingly superficial— are indeed tools, supported by advanced science and utilize naturally occurring substances to enhance the natural beauty of everyone that walks through the doors. Each body is a divinely created canvas—and if given enough care, can ultimately express this unique and natural beauty, even further. This process of enhancement often provides additional confidence and contentment that allows people to actualize—and become—the ideal version of themselves; rather than, a cookie cutter version that media overproduces as "the norm."

As a result of believing the importance in this, I have begun writing a second book that explores how addressing one's lifestyle, in addition to health and fitness, can miraculously transform one's drive and a sense of purpose on this planet. Writing has become an integral part of my mark and legacy that I chose to bestow upon this world. As part of my pursuit toward enjoying life to its fullest, I have fun participating in board sports with my husband—including snowboarding, surfing, and longboarding at Portland's waterfront. Also, as self-proclaimed foodies and wine enthusiasts, we look for any opportunity to partake in Oregon's abundance. And, of course, I can be found investigating new ways to live a minimalistic (or intentional) lifestyle, on a regular basis. But, you figured that, didn't you?

As part of my career, I enjoy teaching in every capacity and am available to guest speak, create topic-specific seminars tailored to you or your company's needs and provide individualized patient care and coaching. Feel free to reach out to me as I welcome the opportunity to serve you and assist you in your journey.

Additional Resources

Cookbooks I love:

Nom Nom Paleo

Primal Blue Print Cookbook

Wheat Belly Cookbook

Wild Diet by "Fat Burning Chef" Abel James

YouTube Documentary to Watch:

https://www.youtube.com/watch?v=QLoXZ-p9OlE (TITLE: Sugar Documentary: How calories from Sugar and Starch is Different than Other Calorie Sources)

YouTube Workout Options:

You Are Your Own Gym (HIIT training and calisthenics)

Sadie Nardini (yoga and HIIT)

Fitness Blender (HIIT, cardio kickboxing, circuit training, body weight and strength training, etc.)

GymRa

BeFit (dance, yoga, HIIT, conditioning training, weight training, etc.)

Tone It Up

Bodyrock (a lot of intense; but, modifiable circuit training and HIIT training)

Blogilates (Cassey Ho has a lot of great pilates-inspired cardio and resistance training videos)

Jessica Smith TV (Total Body Sculpting Resistance Band workout)

Beyoncé "Move Your Body" Full Workout Routine or "Who Run the World" Beyoncé Dance Workout With Benjamin Allen

Tara Stiles: Yoga Weight-Loss & Balance Workout

Yoga With Adriene

Yoga with Kassandra (lots of yin yoga and restorative yoga)

Websites I visit often:

marksdailyapple.com (see free recipe resources and great health advice on this site)

mercola.com (for relevant health information, nutritional guidance, and exercise training)

drhyman.com (for general health information)

journeytowardjoy.com (I have a bias of course)

DoYouYoga.com (for some free and beginner-friendly yoga classes as well as for streaming yoga workouts)

FatBurningMan.com

LesMills.com (for streaming workouts)

beachbody.com (for streaming workouts)

dailyburn.com (for streaming workouts)

YogaGlo.com (for streaming yoga exercises)

physique57.com (for streaming intense barre workouts)

Booya Fitness (for streaming workouts)

Pinterest (for "ketogenic recipes")

https://tim.blog (Tim Ferriss)

Workout DVD's I love:

You Are Your Own Gym (body weight and HIIT training)

Core Strength Vinyasa Yoga by Sadie Nardini (she has four downloadable DVDs available on her website: sadienardini.com).

Physique 57 (pilates and ballet inspired, similar to most barre workouts)

Les Mills Combat (A beachbody.com program) "Ultimate Fighter" series contains HIIT workouts, abdominal training, and mixed martial arts

PiYo Strength kit (A beachbody.com program) A challenging mix of pilates, yoga, cardiovascular training, etc. using body weight)

Les Mills Pump (for practical weight training without a gym; can be done with hand weights or barbell. The DVD series includes an excellent 20-minute yoga flow workout, as well)

Focus T25 (A beachbody.com program — challenging 25 minute HIIT workouts)

Books I Find Useful:

Body By You by Mark Lauren (body weight and calisthenic training for women)

Primal Blue Print by Mark Sisson

Wheat Belly by William Davis, M.D.

Salt, Sugar, Fat by Michael Moss

Grain Brain by Dr. Perlmutter, M.D.

Pounds and Inches by Dr. A.T.W. Simeons (manuscript on the original science behind the hCG diet)

The Art and Science of Low Carbohydrate Living by Stephen D. Phinney and Jeff S. Volek

The Art and Science of Low Carbohydrate Performance by
Stephen D. Phinney and Jeff S. Volek
Jumping For Health by Dr. Morton Walker, M.D.
The Four Hour Body by Timothy Ferriss

Phone Apps that I Use to Track Progress:

My Fitness Pal (for tracking carbohydrate, calorie, macronutrient
intake, logging workouts, etc.)
Cronometer (for tracking the same as My Fitness Pal)
Fat2Fit (to calculate your Body Mass Index, Basal Metabolic Rate,
approximate body fat percentage, etc.)
Heart Math (to provide feedback on resting heart variability, reactions to foods, managing stress better, etc.)

Phone Apps For Weight Loss:

Surf City Apps LLC - The apps to check out: Lose Weight, Enjoy
Exercise, Eat Heathy, Mindful Eating, Sleep Well (you can get
them in a bundle for $10.99) or you can get each individually for
free. I suggest getting one to start with for free, then if you want to
have the "Pro" features of being able to turn off the instructions or
automatic "wake" feature at the end, then you will want to purchase the app for $2.99 each. But try them free first.

YouTube Guided Meditations I Find Useful:

Barry Eisen: Weight Control (13 minutes)
Michael Sealey: Weight Loss (46 minutes) or Weight Loss and
Low Carbohydrate Diets (16 minutes)

Jason Stephenson: Weight Loss meditation (24 minutes) and Top 20 Affirmations for Weight Loss (20 minutes)

GabrielMethodVideo: Visualization for Weight Loss (12 minutes)

Gabriel Method: Nighttime meditation (20 minutes)

Other Resources:

Computer program "f.lux" (for blocking blue screen)

brain fm (app for focus and sleep)

Bullet Proof Food Sense app (to determine food sensitivities)

iThlete (for heart rate variability)

Bioforce app (for heart rate variability)

HRV4Training app (for heart rate variability)

Inner Balance (for heart rate variability)

Sleep Cycle app (monitors quality of sleep and gently wakes you at ideal time)

Sleep Time app (monitors quality of sleep, gently wakes you at ideal time)

vitalchoice.com for home delivery of grass fed meat and safe seafood

Amazon Fresh for home delivery of fresh fruit and vegetable juices

Recommended Tests to Discuss With Your Provider:

Liver detoxification tests: urinary D-glucaric acid and mercapturic acid to test phase I and phase II detoxification pathways.

Oxidative Stress Test: measures how well your body handles free radical stress. PHARMASAN Laboratories is one that I like.

Intestinal Permeability Test: lactulose and mannitol urinary test to measure permeability.

Comprehensive Digestive Stool Analysis (CDSA): to check the "ecosystem" of your gut and determine if there are any unwelcome guests and how well you are digesting food.

Food Sensitivity Testing: Most people with an actual allergy (IgE) have severe reactions to certain foods and know to avoid them. For everyone else, food sensitivity (IgG) s helpful to determine what foods to avoid.

Nutritional Status

Hormone and Adrenal Tests: DUTCH laboratories provides a metabolic breakdown of hormones and cortisol and is very useful. Great Smokies Diagnostic Laboratory now has a hormone test for the public using their website: www.gsdl.com.

Neurotransmitter Tests: PHARMASAN Laboratories has a useful test (that tests hormones and adrenal as well) to determine if neuro-transmitters are deficient or too high and causing weight-related concerns.

Tests You May Order Yourself

Genova Diagnostics (gdx.net) for at-home hormonal evaluation
savonlabs.com for food sensitivity evaluation
mymedialab.com for a variety of laboratory tests
Life Extension for comprehensive hormone blood tests

MY CONTACT INFORMATION:

Dr. Linné Linder

Naturopathic Physician

e-mail: drlinder@journeytowardjoy.com

Facebook: Linné Linder

YouTube: Linné Linder

Instagram: l.linder

Pinterest: Linné Linder

LinkedIn: Linné Linder

webpage/blog: www.journeytowardjoy.com

Notes

My Weight Loss Journey

Sisson, M. (2009). *The Primal Blueprint: Reprogram your genes for effortless weight loss, vibrant health, and boundless energy.* California: Primal Nutrition, Inc.

Your Mindset Determines Your Success

Bandura, A. (2004) "Health Promotion by Social-Cognitive Theory." *Health Education and Behavior.* (vol. 31, 143-164)

Barling, J. & Abel, M (1983) "Self-Efficacy Beliefs and Performance." *Cognitive Theory and Research.* (Vol 7, 265-272).

Locke, E.A., & Latham, G.P. (1984) *Goal Setting: A Motivational Technique that Works.* Englewood Cliffs, NJ: Prentice-Hall.

Niemark, J. (1987) "The Power of Positive Thinkers. " Reprinted from *Success Magazine*, September 1987.

Weight Loss is About Calories and Activity, Right?

D'Eon, T. & Braun, B. (2002) "The Roles of Estrogen and Progesterone in Regulating Carbohydrate and Fat Utilization at Rest and During Exercise." *Journal of Women's Health and Gender-Based Medicine* 11no. 3, 225-37

Kuo, L.E., Czarnecka, M., Kitlinska, J.B., Tilan, J.U., Kvetnansky, R. & Zukowska, Z. (Dec. 2008) "Chronic Stress, Combined with a High-Fat/High-Sugar Diet, Shifts Sympathetic Signaling toward

Neuropeptide Y and Leads to Obesity and the Metabolic Syndrome." *Annals of the New York Academy of Sciences* 1148, 232-7. don: 10.7326/0003-4819-153-3-201008030-00005.

Meraglia, T. (2015). *The Hormone Secret: Discover Effortless Weight Los and Renewed Energy in Just 30 Days.* New York: Atria Books.

Teta, J. & Teta, K. (2015) *Lose Weight Here.* New York: Rodale.

Teta, J & Teta, K. (2010) *The Metabolic Effect Diet: Eat More, Work Out Less, and Actually Lose Weight While You Rest.* New York: HarperCollins.

Tremblay, A., Royer, M.M., Chalut, J.P. & Doucet, E. (2013) "Adaptive Thermogenesis Can Make a Difference in the Ability of Obese Individuals to Lose Body Weight." *International Journal of Obesity* 37, 759-64.

The Plan: Approved Foods

Garaulet, M., Gómez-Abellán, P.et al., (2013) "Timing of food intake predicts weight loss effectiveness," *International Journal of Obesity*: 37, 604-611/doi.10.1038/ijo.2012.229.

Teta, J. (2012, March). *How to Stop Food Cravings: Understanding Trigger and Buffer Foods.* Retrieved from http://www. metaboliceffect.com/how-to-stop-food-cravings.

The Plan: Creating Your Workout Routine

Bryner, R.W, Ullrich, I.H., Sauers, J., Donley, D., Hornsby, G., Kolar, M. & Yeater, R. (Apr. 1999) "Effects of Resistance vs. Aerobic Training Combines with an 800 Calorie Liquid Diet on Lean Body Mass and Resting Metabolic Rate." *Journal of the American College of Nutrition* 18, no. 2, 115-21.

Hansen, D., Dendale, P., Berger, J., van Loon, L.J. & Meeusen, R. (Jan 2007) "The Effects of Exercise Training on Fat-Mass Loss in Obese Patients During energy Intake Restriction." *Sports Medicine* 37, no. 1, 31-46.

Hughes, J.; Fresco, D.; Myerscough, R., et al., (2013) "Randomized Controlled Trial of Mindfulness-Based Stress Reduction for Prehypertension," *Psychosomatic Medicine* vol. 75 no. 9, 721-729.

Sanjay R. Patel, Atul Malhotra, et al., (2006) "Association Between Reduced Sleep and Weight Gain in Women," *American Journal of Epidemiology,* 164 (10), 947-954.

Daily Detoxification
Batmanghelidj, F. (2008). *Your Body's Many Cries for Water.* Virginia: Global Health Solutions.
Walker, M. (2011). *Jumping for Health.* New York: KE Publishing.

Recipes
Tam, M. & Fong, H. *Nom Nom Paleo Food For Humans.* Missouri: Andrews McMeel Publishing, LL

Monica

Made in the USA
San Bernardino, CA
29 June 2019